☑ **W9-BYA-626**

WITHDRAWN

7+3
10/23/06

5+1
11/13/04

New Canaan Library

151 Main Street
New Canaan, CT 06840

(203)594-5000
www.newcanaanlibrary.org

DEMCO

AUG 28 2003

Books published by the American Cancer Society

A Breast Cancer Journey: Your Personal Guidebook

American Cancer Society's Complementary and Alternative Cancer Methods Handbook

American Cancer Society's Guide to Complementary and Alternative Cancer Methods

American Cancer Society's Guide to Pain Control

Angels & Monsters: A Child's Eye View of Cancer, Murray and Howard

Because Someone I Love Has Cancer: Kids' Activity Book

Cancer in the Family: Helping Children Cope with a Parent's Illness, Heiney et al.

Caregiving: A Step-By-Step Resource for Caring for the Person with Cancer at Home, Houts and Bucher

Colorectal Cancer: A Thorough and Compassionate Resource for Patients and Their Families, Levin

Coming to Terms with Cancer: A Glossary of Cancer-Related Terms, Laughlin

Consumers Guide to Cancer Drugs, Wilkes, Ades, and Krakoff

Couples Confronting Cancer: Keeping Your Relationship Strong, Fincannon and Bruss

Crossing Divides: A Couple's Story of Cancer, Hope, and Hiking Montana's Continental Divide, Bischke

Good for You! Reducing Your Risk of Developing Cancer

Informed Decisions: The Complete Book of Cancer Diagnosis, Treatment, and Recovery, 2nd Edition, Eyre, Lange, and Morris

Kicking Butts: Your Path to Quitting Smoking

Our Mom Has Cancer, Ackermann and Ackermann

Prostate Cancer: What Every Man—and His Family—Needs to Know, Revised Edition, Bostwick et al.

Women and Cancer: A Thorough and Compassionate Resource for Patients and Their Families, Runowicz, Petrek, and Gansler

Also by the American Cancer Society

American Cancer Society's Healthy Eating Cookbook: A Celebration of Food, Friends, and Healthy Living, 2nd Edition

Celebrate! Healthy Entertaining for Any Occasion

Kids' First Cookbook: Delicious-Nutritious Treats to Make Yourself!

CANCER:
What Causes It,
What Doesn't

FROM THE EXPERTS AT THE
AMERICAN CANCER SOCIETY

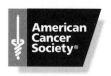

616.994
C

Published by
American Cancer Society
Health Promotions
1599 Clifton Road NE
Atlanta, Georgia 30329, USA

Managing Editor
Gianna Marsella, M.A.

Editor
Amy Sproull Brittain

Copy Editor
Anneke Smith

Contributing Writer
Carol Clark

Editorial Review
Rick Alteri, M.D.
Ted Gansler, M.D., M.B.A.

Managing Director, Direct Channels
Chuck Westbrook

Director, Publishing
Diane Scott-Lichter, M.A.

Book Publishing Manager
Candace Magee

Copyright ©2003 American Cancer Society
All rights reserved. Without limiting the rights
under copyright reserved above, no part of this
publication may be reproduced, stored in or
introduced into a retrieval system, or transmitted, in any form or by any means (electronic,
mechanical, photocopying, recording, or other-
wise), without the prior written permission of
the publisher.

Printed in the United States of America
Cover designed by Jill Dible, Atlanta, GA

5 4 3 2 1   03 04 05 06 07

Library of Congress Cataloging-in-Publication Data

Cancer : what causes it, what doesn't.
      p. ; cm.
  ISBN 0-944235-44-1 (pbk. : alk. paper)
  1. Cancer--Risk factors--Popular works. 2. Cancer--Etiology--Popular
works.
    [DNLM: 1. Neoplasms--etiology--Popular Works. 2.
Neoplasms--genetics--Popular Works. QZ 201 C2149 2003] I. American
Cancer Society.

RC263.C298 2003
616.99'4071--dc21

                                        2003001116

A NOTE TO THE READER
The information contained in this book is not intended as medical advice and should
not be relied upon as a substitute for talking with your doctor. This information may
not address all possible actions, precautions, side effects, or interactions. All matters
regarding your health require the supervision of a medical doctor who is familiar
with your medical needs. For more information, contact your American Cancer
Society at 800-ACS-2345 (www.cancer.org).

Contents

Introduction

CAN YOU GET CANCER FROM DEODORANT, talcum powder, or cellular phones? Which cancer "risks" should you be concerned about and which are just rumors? What do your everyday activities and genetic makeup have to do with your personal cancer risk? How does cancer start and why?

No one book can draw a complete picture of cancer—cancer has perplexed humans for at least 5,000 years. Researchers discover new information at such a fast pace that it would be a challenge for anyone to absorb it all. It seems that the more answers we find, the more questions we raise.

But this book shares much of what we know about the how and why of cancer. As we dispel myths, explain risks, and explore the ins and outs of cancer, we hope you'll gain valuable understanding about cancer, what causes it, and what doesn't.

Information Overload

Cancer is in the headlines every day. Unsubstantiated rumors about cancer hitch a ride on the Internet and rocket around the world in a matter of hours. Daily news articles report on the potential risks of ordinary substances we come into contact with, frightening us and making us rethink our choices.

People shouldn't panic when they hear that a new study shows a substance causes cancer in mice—nor should they believe they are immune from cancer because they eat well and exercise regularly, advises C. Everett Koop, M.D., former U.S. Surgeon General and director of the Koop Institute at Dartmouth Medical School in Hanover, New Hampshire.

"When you concentrate on the wrong information about cancer, you don't do the right things that could save your life," Koop says.

This book will help you concentrate on the *right* information. We'll clear up some common misconceptions about the causes of cancer and give you the facts you need to know about cancer risks you inherit and those you can control.

Find Out the Real Risks

Compelling reports about the role of genetics in cancer, the effects of powerful environmental *carcinogens* (chemicals and other exposures that cause cancer), and the possibility of radiation leaks from nuclear power plants sometimes obscure a key cancer issue: *Two-thirds of all fatal cancers are associated with lifestyle choices.* So while some cancer risks are out of your hands, some are squarely in your control. Factors as basic as what you eat and drink can affect your cancer risk.

"We really have an enormous amount of control over our risks," says Eugenia Calle, Ph.D., the American Cancer Society's director of analytic epidemiology. "If everybody maintained a lean body mass, didn't smoke, ate a lot of fruits and vegetables, protected their skin from the sun, and exercised every day, we would live in a different society. It doesn't mean that cancer would be gone. But it would have a huge, huge impact on the rates of cancer."

Cancer: Past, Present, and Future

Today cancer is a disease that can often be diagnosed early and treated successfully, allowing more and more people to call themselves cancer survivors. But even before we had a name for cancer, it was claiming lives.

In chapter 1, we retrace the history of our struggle to understand cancer, from the mysticism of ancient Egypt to the many new directions molecular science is taking. We'll relive the dramatic discoveries that have saved lives and that have implications for discoveries still to come.

In chapter 2, we clarify who is at risk for cancer, expose how scientists gather information about cancer in certain populations, and discuss how demographic factors (like age, race, and socioeconomic status) affect your cancer risk.

We travel inside the cellular structures of DNA in chapter 3 to reveal how cancer develops and what role genetics and family history play in cancer.

The information in chapter 4 will help you make sense of scientific studies and allow you to become a more informed consumer of medical research.

Environmental hazards like radiation and pesticides are discussed in chapter 5—along with information on whether you really need to worry about them. Chapter 6 tackles cancer risks you might encounter while at home and on the job.

Chapter 7 reveals that most cancers can be prevented by making healthy lifestyle choices, like eating right, staying active, and cutting out tobacco.

Finally, we conclude with a discussion of what the future may hold for cancer research.

In just the last 50 years, we've uncovered most of what we know about what causes cancer, revolutionizing our ability to screen, diagnose, and treat cancer, and saving hundreds of thousands of lives. Just imagine what discoveries the next 50 years will bring.

CHAPTER 1

From Mummies to Molecular Genetics

I N THE SUMMER OF 1953, Anne Talley was preparing for her wedding. The 21-year-old native of Memphis, Tennessee, had just graduated from college and was engaged to Irvin Fleming, another young Memphis native about to enter medical school.

For weeks, Talley had occasionally felt a nagging pain in her left arm. "When something would hit my arm accidentally, I felt some pain but not enough to stop all my activities," she says. Two weeks before her wedding date, Talley fell and fractured her left humerus. The emergency room x-rays revealed why her bone was so weak—a large malignant tumor was growing in it. She had what was then called reticulum cell sarcoma (now known as *non-Hodgkin's lymphoma*), a cancer of the blood-forming organs that is linked to problems with the body's immune system.

Chemotherapy was not available at that time and Talley had only one viable treatment option—amputation of her arm, all the way up to her shoulder socket. She underwent the surgery and two weeks later, Anne Talley and Irvin Fleming got married. "I was released from the hospital on a Wednesday, and I was married on a Saturday," she says. "My wedding dress was kind of high necked, but you could see the bandage through the lace and I just tied the left arm up. It was kind of dramatic."

Today non-Hodgkin's lymphoma of the bone can be treated with chemotherapy and radiation therapy instead of surgery. But researchers still do not know what causes it, or why incidences of it have been increasing through the years.

Meanwhile, Anne and Irvin Fleming are looking forward to their fiftieth wedding anniversary. She keeps busy as a dog show judge. Irvin Fleming, M.D., a past president of the American Cancer Society (ACS), is now a professor of surgery at the University of Tennessee and the director of the Methodist HealthCare Cancer Center in Memphis.

He is hopeful that with the explosion of new cancer detection and research technologies, valuable insights about non-Hodgkin's lymphoma and other types of cancer will be gained soon. "We're on the threshold of a new research approach, based on a lot of new genetic information that is coming out," Fleming says. "It's a whole new science that's developing."

Cancer in the Ancient World

Anne Fleming's story illustrates how far we've come in the past few decades, and how much scientists have yet to learn about what causes cancer. But cancer is not only a recent concern. The mysteries of cancer have plagued humans for at least the past five millennia. Although we now know that *cancer* is a group of diseases that causes cells in the body to change and grow out of control, the desire to understand the deadly disease exceeded our predecessors' limited knowledge about the human body. In order to come to terms with the unknown, they developed many theories about what causes cancer.

Cancer Goes on Record

The ancient Egyptians recorded their medical knowledge and left behind surgical handbooks, outlines for medical lectures, and case notes on papyrus manuscripts. Two ancient papyri, written about 1600 B.C. but believed to date from sources as early as 2500 B.C., describe surgical, pharmacological, and magical treatments for cancer. These records are the first known documentations of cancer.

Ancient Egyptians believed supernatural forces caused illnesses like cancer. Rosalie David, Ph.D., a *paleopathologist* and keeper of Egyptology at the Manchester Museum, notes, "Ancient Egyptian medicine was sophisticated, but they mixed rational methods with magic — the two went side by side. If they couldn't see the obvious cause of an internal disease, they often attributed it to evil spirits, the bad wishes of your enemies, or even to the powers of the dead."

In addition to their medical records, the ancient Egyptians provided modern cancer researchers with another legacy — their own bodies. In an effort to achieve immortality, the pharaohs of ancient Egypt were embalmed. Some of the earliest evidence of cancer has been found in the remains of these mummies.

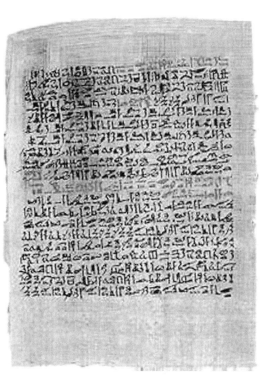

Two ancient Egyptian papyri that describe cancer were discovered and deciphered in the 1800s. Image courtesy of the National Cancer Institute.

Unwrapping the
Medical Mysteries of Mummies

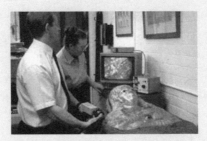

Studying mummies helps modern scientists
learn about ancient diseases. Photo courtesy
of The Manchester Museum, University of
Manchester.

Egyptologists and forensic specialists at the Manchester Museum in
Manchester, England, are unwrapping the medical mysteries of mum-
mies to trace the ancient history of a disease known as *schistosomiasis*.
Urinary schistosomiasis, left untreated, can lead to bladder cancer.

Schistosomiasis is caused by a type of flatworm called a fluke that
penetrates the skin of swimmers in the Nile River. People can also
become infected by drinking contaminated water. The worms grow
inside a human's blood vessels and produce eggs that can travel to different parts of the body, damaging the liver, intestines, lungs, and
bladder. One ancient papyrus describes the symptoms of urinary
schistosomiasis and attributes these symptoms to a disease called *aaa*.

Using modern forensic and clinical techniques that enable scientists
to analyze small samples of tissue and leave the mummies intact,
researchers have been able to detect the fluke worms that cause urinary
schistosomiasis in the urinary and bladder tissue of ancient mummies,
says Rosalie David, Ph.D., who also directs the Schistosomiasis
Investigation Project.

Researchers will compile the data extracted from mummies with
data about current schistosomiasis cases in Africa, where the modern-
day incidence of bladder cancer can be up to 32 times higher than the
rate of bladder cancer in the United States. By examining how schistosomiasis has developed over the past 5,000 years, researchers hope
to gain new insights into the links between schistosomiasis and cancer.

The Black Bile Theory

After the decline of the Egyptian empire, the great doctors of Greece and Rome became powerful forces in medicine. The Greek physician Hippocrates, known as "the Father of Medicine," recorded cases of malignant tumors of the breast, uterus, stomach, skin, and mouth in about 400 B.C. He named this condition *karkinoma*, Greek for "crab-like growth." Modern physicians use the term *carcinoma* to refer to malignant tumors that grow in the tissue that covers or lines external and internal body surfaces.

Hippocrates' approach to medicine was based on the theory that the human body was composed of four humors, or body fluids—blood, phlegm, yellow bile, and black bile—that affected a person's health. These body humors were the biological counterparts of the four elements—air, fire, earth, and water. His theory held that an imbalance in these four humors caused diseases. Cancer was believed to be the result of an excess of black bile, curable only in its earliest stages.

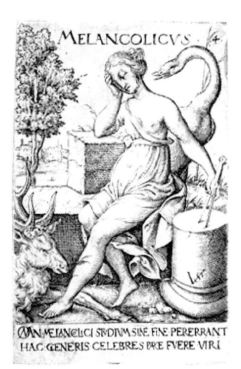

The Roman physician Galen was probably the most influential figure in medicine from the Roman Empire to the Renaissance. Galen wrote over 400 works on a huge range of medical topics; many of these treatises were still considered authoritative 1500 years later. Like Hippocrates, Galen believed that cancer was caused by an excess of black bile. He gave fleshy tumors the name *sarcoma* (fleshy growth). Today, physicians use the same term to describe malignant tumors arising in the connective tissues.

Individuals with an excess of black bile were called melancholic. The modern term "melancholy" comes from this ancient medical theory. Photographic reproduction of an engraving of Melancolicus 4 Virgilius Solis, the Elder (1514–1562) courtesy of the National Library of Medicine.

Foundations of Modern Science

The Seventeenth Century: Lymphatic Origins

The theory of disease based on the body's four humors prevailed in Western medicine until the 1600s, when researchers began looking for other explanations for cancer. Gaspare Aselli's discovery of the *lymphatic system* (the tissues and vessels that create, store, and transport white blood cells to fight infection) led to the idea that cancer arose from an abnormality in *lymph*, the clear fluid that contains white blood cells.

The Eighteenth Century: Environmental Insights

In the eighteenth century, some historically important observations were made about environmental causes of cancer.

In the mid 1700s, John Hill of London linked the development of nasal polyps to the habit of inhaling tobacco. Hill published a report condemning snuff, writing, "No man should venture upon snuff, who is not sure that he is not so far liable to cancer: and no man can be sure of that."

In 1775, Percival Pott, a surgeon at London's St. Bartholomew's Hospital, reported that overexposure to soot was causing cancer of the scrotum in young chimney sweeps. Pott felt great compassion for the young men he observed, many of whom began working as children, when they were small enough to fit into the chimneys. "The fate of these people seems singularly hard...they are thrust up narrow, and sometimes hot chimnies [*sic*], where they are bruised, burned, and almost suffocated; and then they get to puberty, become peculiarly liable to a most noisome, painful, and fatal disease," Pott wrote.

In 1795, Samuel Thomas von Soemmering, a Polish professor of anatomy living in Germany, noted: "Carcinoma of the lip is most frequent when people indulge in tobacco pipes. For the lower lip is particularly attacked by carcinoma because it is compressed between the pipe and the teeth."

The Nineteenth Century: Knowledge Advances

The reversal of bans against autopsy and dissection allowed for the development of *morbid* or *pathological anatomy* (the study of the structural changes in the body that accompany disease). Early illustrated pathology textbooks provided detailed descriptions of cancers of the breast, stomach, rectum, testes, bladder, pancreas, and esophagus.

Technological advancements in this century sparked many exciting scientific inventions, including better microscopes. Johannes Müller, dean of the faculty at the University of Berlin, began the study of tumors under the microscope in 1836. His 1838 book established that tumors are composed of disorganized abnormal cells. Müller's work introduced *histology* (the study of tissue) and revealed that cells of cancerous tumors were different from the cells of normal surrounding tissue.

Medical demography (the statistical study of human populations to understand disease patterns) first began in the 1600s; by the mid-1800s, analysis of cancer statistics collected in France and Italy resulted in several important findings. Domenico Rigoni-Stern reported that cancer rates increased with age, cancer occurred more often in urban environments, and unmarried people were more likely to develop the disease.

More instances of cancers linked to specific occupations were noted as the industrial revolution got underway. A high rate of lung cancer among miners of Germany's Black Forest was described in 1879, and aniline dye industry workers were reported to be at high risk for cancer of the bladder in 1895.

Konrad Wilhelm Roentgen discovered x-rays and their unique properties in 1895, and Pierre and Marie Curie identified radium in 1898. Both discoveries led to the development of important tools for cancer detection and therapy.

It wasn't until several decades later, in 1928, that scientists realized the carcinogenic effects of radium. Young girls employed in factories painting radium dials on watches were found to have high rates of various types of cancers. The cause was traced back to the girls' habit of using their tongues to sharpen the tips of their paintbrushes. Studies of survivors of atomic bombs dropped in World War II would later provide definitive evidence of the carcinogenic effects of radiation.

Into the Modern Age

Discovering Cancer Causes

The early twentieth century saw several new discoveries about the origins of cancer. Scientists confirmed chromosomal, viral, and chemical causes of cancer.

In the early 1900s, Theodor Boveri, a German professor of zoology, advocated the theory that cancer was due to abnormalities in *chromosomes*, the microscopic structures that transmit hereditary information. This theory would come to the forefront decades later with the rise of molecular genetics.

Viruses are very small disease-causing organisms that are unable to reproduce without a host cell. An American researcher named Peyton Rous isolated a virus in 1911 that caused tumors to develop in chickens, but the microscopes available at the time were not powerful enough to make the virus visible. Rous' discovery went relatively unrecognized until the invention of the electron microscope 50 years later.

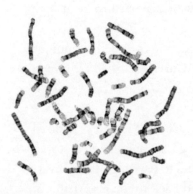 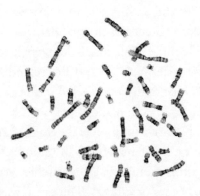

The chromosomes of a human male (left), and a human female (right). Image courtesy of the University of Washington Department of Pathology, *http://www.pathology.washington.edu/galleries/cytogallery/cytogallery.html.*

New experimental techniques in the twentieth century also allowed researchers to show conclusively that certain chemicals could cause cancer in animals. Despite such advances, misinformation still abounded. The idea that cancer was caused by physical trauma was still common through the 1920s, even though experiments on animals showed no link between cancer and physical injury.

Cancer's Public Profile

Cancer moved out of the laboratory and into the public realm in 1913 with the publication of an article on cancer's warning signs in a popular women's magazine.

That same year, the American Society for the Control of Cancer (later renamed the American Cancer Society) was founded. In the beginning, the society's sole mission was to educate the public and physicians about cancer, although it later expanded into research as well.

One of the founders of the society was an insurance statistician named Frederik Hoffman. At his urging, the U.S. Census Bureau compiled its first analysis of cancer mortality data in 1914. The following year, Hoffman published an analysis of global cancer statistics.

As Americans enjoyed increasingly longer lifestyles, and infectious diseases became less of a threat, fighting chronic diseases such as cancer became a higher priority for the U.S. public health system. In 1937, Congress made conquering cancer a national goal, unanimously passing an act establishing the National Cancer Institute.

The Tobacco Watershed

The practice of inhaling burning tobacco leaves started at least 2500 years ago in Central America, where the Mayans attributed healing powers to the practice. The myth of tobacco's medicinal properties continued with its introduction to Europe at the end of the 1400s. Tobacco was chewed, inhaled as a powder, or applied locally to treat coughs, asthma, headaches, stomach cramps, and malignant tumors, among other maladies.

Evidence of tobacco's harmful effects accumulated slowly beginning in the 1700s. Small studies and observations kept hinting at the association of tobacco with cancers of the lip, mouth, esophagus, and lungs, but none of them provided definitive proof. Meanwhile, smoking grew into a widespread practice as the technology evolved to mass produce cigarettes and distribute them.

In 1950, four major studies published in the United States concluded that lung cancer was associated with smoking. This watershed event in cancer research created little more than a ripple at the time.

The evidence against tobacco kept mounting as studies continued in the United States and other countries as well. In 1964, the Surgeon General of the United States issued a report on smoking and health, over heavy tobacco industry opposition. By 1966, warnings of health risks appeared on cigarette packages.

In 1986, a landmark report was published by the U.S. Surgeon General on the association between *environmental tobacco smoke (ETS)*, also called *secondhand smoke*, and adverse health effects on nonsmokers. The report concluded that ETS can cause lung cancer in healthy adult nonsmokers and that the children of parents who smoke have more respiratory symptoms and evidence of reduced lung function.

Looking back on his long career, Sir Richard Doll, M.D., an *epidemiologist* (a scientist who studies the causes, distribution, and control of disease in populations), recalls many swings in society's perceptions about the causes of cancer. "For a period in the 1970s and early 1980s, there was a perception that the chemical industry was responsible for a large proportion of cancers," he says. "There was also a time when infections and viruses were believed to be the main cause of cancer. Indeed, they are the cause of some cancers, but not of all of them."

Due to this confusion, the U.S. Congress in 1981 commissioned Doll and his colleague, Sir Richard Peto, to quantify U.S. cancer risk factors from a variety of environmental contributions. After reviewing all of the accumulated evidence, Doll and Peto produced a groundbreaking report called *The Causes of Cancer: Quantitative Estimates of Avoidable Risks of Cancer in the United States Today.*

They estimated that tobacco use and dietary choices accounted for two thirds of fatal cancers, while workplace exposures accounted for only 4 percent of cancer deaths and manmade pollution a mere 2 percent.

"The report was very important because it had a lot of immediate policy implications in terms of what we should focus on if we want to prevent cancer," says Mark Parascandola, Ph.D., M.P.H., a cancer prevention fellow at the National Cancer Institute in Bethesda, Maryland. "We still refer to the figures in it today."

Cancer Today

While *epidemiology* (the branch of medicine that studies the causes, distribution, and control of disease in populations) made tremendous strides during the last half century, *molecular biology* (the branch of science devoted to studying the structure, function, and reactions of molecules involved in life processes) also came of age as scientists developed the technology to observe subatomic particles and process information about them.

Looking Inward for Answers

By the middle of the twentieth century, scientists had in their hands the instruments needed to begin solving the mysteries of cancer. In 1953, James Watson and Francis Crick revealed the structure of *deoxyribonucleic acid (DNA)*, the cellular material that contains genetic information. An explosion of discoveries about the different parts of cells and how they function soon followed.

DNA was found to be the basis of the genetic code that gives orders to all cells. After learning how to translate this code, scientists were able to understand how *genes* (segments of DNA that control the expression of traits) worked and how they could be damaged by *mutations* (changes or mistakes in cells). These modern advances in chemistry and biology answered many complex questions about cancer.

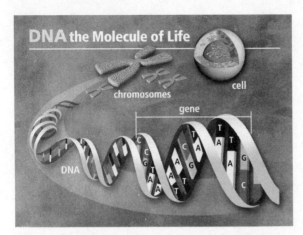

DNA the Molecule of Life

chromosomes

cell

gene

DNA

Cells are the fundamental units of every living system. All the instructions needed to direct cellular activities are contained within DNA. Image courtesy of the Oak Ridge National Laboratory.

Scientists already knew that cancer could be caused by chemicals, radiation, and viruses, and that sometimes cancer seemed to run in families. But, as our understanding of DNA and genes increased, scientists learned that it was the damage to DNA by chemicals and radiation or introduction of new DNA sequences by viruses that often led to the development of cancer. In some cases it became possible to pinpoint the exact site of the damage to a specific gene.

Furthermore, scientists discovered that normal cells with damaged DNA normally die, but cancer cells manage to survive with damaged DNA. The recent discovery of this critical difference answers many questions that have troubled scientists for years.

Mapping the Human Genome

The mapping and cataloguing of the human *genome*—the total genetic material contained within an organism—has set the stage for gaining far deeper insights into the complex causes of cancer as we enter the twenty-first century.

In their careful study of the 30,000 genes that each of us carries, scientists are identifying the genes that are damaged by chemicals or radiation and the gene mutations that, when inherited, can lead to cancer. The recent discovery of two gene mutations that cause some breast cancers is exciting, because many people who have a higher probability of developing breast cancer can now be identified.

Other genes have been discovered that are associated with some cancers that run in families, such as cancers of the colon, rectum,

The Human Genome Project

The Human Genome Project is an international effort formally begun in October 1990. The project was projected to last 15 years, but rapid technological advances accelerated the expected completion date to 2003. Project goals are to discover the approximately 30,000 human genes, determine the complete sequence of the 3 billion or so DNA chemical base pairs that make up human DNA, and make them accessible for further biological study. An additional goal is to address the ethical, legal, and social issues that may arise from the project.

As part of the Human Genome Project, scientists are conducting parallel studies on selected organisms such as the bacterium *E. coli* to help refine gene-mapping technologies and to interpret human gene function. The Department of Energy's Human Genome Program and the National Institutes of Health's National Human Genome Research Institute together make up the U.S. Human Genome Project.

Several types of genome maps have already been completed, and a rough draft of the entire human genome sequence was announced in June 2000. First analyses were published in February 2001. Efforts are still underway to complete the finished, high-quality sequence.

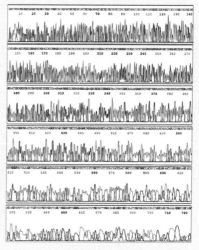

Genome Sequence Trace. Image courtesy of the Oak Ridge National Laboratory.

kidney, ovary, esophagus, lymph nodes, pancreas, and skin. Such cases of familial cancer are not nearly as common as spontaneous (non-inherited) cancer, which accounts for nearly 85 percent of all cancers. But understanding inherited cancers provides vital information to scientists about what causes cancer on a molecular level.

What Lies Ahead

The growth in our knowledge of cancer biology and cancer treatment and prevention has been staggering in recent years. Scientists and *oncologists* (doctors who specialize in the treatment of cancer) have learned more about cancer in the last decade of the twentieth century than in all the centuries preceding.

Despite these amazing advances, huge gaps remain in our understanding of cancer. Although we are rapidly exposing cancer's secrets, the knowledge we gain continuously brings up new questions and new avenues to explore.

Says Robert Weinberg, Ph.D., from the Whitehead Institute of Biomedical Research in Cambridge, Massachusetts, "We've only begun to scratch the surface."

CHAPTER 2

Who Is at Risk for Cancer?

HAROLD FREEMAN, M.D., AN AFRICAN AMERICAN, was born in Washington, D.C., to a family with little money but a lot of ambition. His mother was an elementary school teacher and his father struggled to become a lawyer, attending classes while working odd jobs like driving a cab. His father finally got his law degree at age 43, but just six years later he died of testicular cancer.

Freeman was 13 years old then and had two older brothers. His mother raised the boys on a schoolteacher's salary.

His father's death had a profound impact on Freeman's future career. When he later became a surgeon, he chose oncology as his specialty, completing his training in 1967. He decided to work in Harlem, New York.

"Harlem is a poor, black neighborhood, and I had a sense I should use my training and skills in such a neighborhood," he says. "I thought that was where I could have the biggest impact."

Freeman was struck by the extraordinarily poor cancer outcomes for Harlem patients. Most of the breast cancer patients he saw did not come for treatment until they were in an advanced stage of the disease. "I knew there was something different about working in a black community," he recalls.

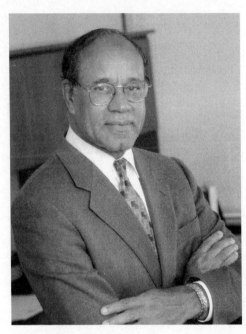

Harold Freeman, M.D.

In 1973, the journal *Cancer* published a landmark report titled "Alarming Increase of the Cancer Mortality in the U.S. Black Population." The article brought to people's attention that blacks were dying of cancer at a higher rate than anyone else in America. Today, the group's death rate from cancer is about 33 percent higher than that of Caucasians. African Americans also have a higher overall rate of cancer than any other ethnic or racial group.

Freeman, a former president of the American Cancer Society (ACS), is chairman of the President's Cancer Panel, director of the National Cancer Institute's Center for Reducing Health Disparities, and chief of surgery at North General Hospital in New York City. Freeman devoted his career to finding out why some segments of the population had higher cancer incidence rates and lower survival rates. As cancer data collection techniques have become more detailed and consistent on a national scale, other researchers have joined the effort.

Understanding Cancer Risk

About one of every two American men and one of every three American women will have some type of cancer at some point during their lifetime. Will you be one of them?

How much of a role do factors beyond our control play in cancer risk? In this chapter, we'll explore what age, race, and socioeconomic status have to do with your risk of developing cancer. We'll also look at how researchers monitor demographic groups to better understand where and why cancer occurs.

Cancer can strike people of all ages, nationalities, and walks of life. Anyone can get cancer, but over three-fourths of all cancers occur in people older than 55. And although cancer occurs in Americans of all racial and ethnic groups, the rate of the development of new cases of cancer (sometimes called the *incidence rate*) varies from group to group.

As researchers sift through statistics on types of cancers, including cancer patients' ages, cultural and ethnic backgrounds, and where they live, they consider questions that may help them figure out why certain groups of people develop cancer, such as:

- Why do most forms of cancer rarely strike people younger than 30 and show a marked increase in occurrence in people older than 50?

- Why are African Americans more likely to develop cancer and die from it than any other race or ethnic group?

- Why does the rate of cancer incidence change in certain populations, such as Asians, after immigration to the United States?

The more we learn about specific cancer patterns, the more we know that no one is immune from the group of complex diseases known as cancer.

Lifetime Probability of Developing Cancer

The following chart shows the chance of an adult in the United States being diagnosed with cancer over the course of a lifetime. The information shows overall data and data for the four most frequently occurring cancers in men and women, based on 1996–1998 incidence data.

Males		Females	
Overall	1 in 2	Overall	1 in 3
Prostate	1 in 6	Breast	1 in 8
Lung and Bronchus	1 in 13	Lung and Bronchus	1 in 17
Colorectal	1 in 17	Colorectal	1 in 18
Bladder	1 in 29	Uterine/Endometrial	1 in 37

Looking for Patterns:
Researchers and Cancer Data

Knowing the effect of age, race, and socioeconomic status on cancer risk requires careful sleuthing. Researchers collect and analyze information about cancer deaths, new cancer cases, extent of the disease, screening tests, treatment, and survival. This is called *cancer surveillance*. Using this cancer data, researchers can identify trends over time, discover cancer patterns among populations, and determine whether screening and other prevention measures are making a difference.

A high cancer incidence rate in one segment of a population is a red flag to epidemiologists, scientists who study the factors that affect patterns of diseases in populations. They try to identify risk factors and pinpoint possible causes of cancer. The more detailed the data and the larger the population surveyed, the more useful cancer data becomes to researchers. In some cases, it's fairly easy for researchers to figure out why one group has a higher rate of a type of cancer than another. In other cases, it's much more difficult.

Data Dateline

Scientists in the United States have gathered statistics on cancer death since the nineteenth century, but collecting patient profiles and detailed data on incidence rates of specific cancers—and then compiling them in cancer registries—is relatively new.

1971: The National Cancer Act of 1971 authorizes the collection, analysis, and distribution of data to help prevent, treat, and diagnose cancer in the United States.

1973: The National Cancer Institute (NCI), the federal government's principal agency for cancer research and training, establishes the Surveillance, Epidemiology and End Results (SEER) Program. The SEER Program collects cancer data from a representative U.S. sample, and the NCI publishes these cancer statistics every year in a report that details incidence and mortality rates, broken down by race, sex, age, and cancer site.

1975: Investigators at the International Agency for Research on Cancer begin using data from other countries to publish comparisons between different nationalities' cancer incidence.

1989: The National Cancer Data Base, jointly supported by the American Cancer Society and the American College of Surgeons Commission on Cancer, is established to collect data to monitor and improve the quality of cancer care.

1992: The Cancer Registries Amendments Act authorizes the creation of the National Program of Cancer Registries (NPCR), a Centers for Disease Control and Prevention (CDC) program. Through the NPCR, the CDC improves, creates, and provides training for cancer registries.

1992: The SEER Program increases coverage of information about minority populations, especially Hispanics.

"Differences in cancer rates for geographic areas and among ethnic groups get researchers interested in the differences in those populations," says Elizabeth Ward, Ph.D., the director of surveillance research for the ACS. She explains that by process of elimination, researchers can sometimes develop theories about what causes cancer.

Just the Facts, Please

A patient's diagnosis and *demographics* (race, age, ethnicity, and socioeconomic status) can be helpful information for researchers studying when and where cancer occurs. *Casefinding*, or identifying people with cancer who have sought care at hospitals and doctor's offices, is the first step in cancer epidemiology, the study of the causes, distribution, and control of cancer in populations. Once cases are identified, patient information is stored in repositories called *cancer registries*. Cancer registries collect information about cancer detection, diagnosis, stage of disease, treatment, and survival, as well as patients' demographics. Government and private organizations then analyze the data in cancer registries to learn more about cancer's effects on specific populations.

The "Graying" of America

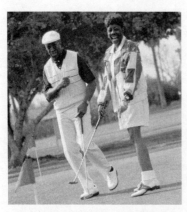

Americans are living longer, healthier lives.

If you are lucky enough to live a long life, you will develop the single highest risk factor for cancer: old age.

People in the United States can look forward to longer lives than ever before. The number of Americans over the age of 65 increased tenfold during the last 100 years, and Americans' average lifespan has increased by 25 years during the past century. Females born today have a life expectancy of 85 years, and males will live an average of 77 years.

In 2011, the first of the 76 million baby boomers will reach the age of 65, launching an era of "elder boomers." By the year 2030, it is estimated that one in four Americans will be over the age of 65.

The aging trend isn't only happening in the United States; it's global in scale. The planet is rapidly approaching a period of unprecedented growth in its older population. By the year 2050, an estimated two billion people will be over the age of 60, which will lead to a huge increase in illnesses associated with aging, including cancer.

As Americans live longer—because of improved health care, healthier diets, and exercise habits—their risk for developing cancer rises. "The good thing in America is we're living longer, but as we get older, we're going to see more cancer," says Hyman Muss, M.D., director of clinical research at the Vermont Cancer Center and a professor of medicine at the University of Vermont in Burlington, Vermont.

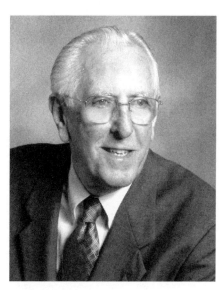

B.J. Kennedy, M.D.

Cancer is primarily a disease of the aging, explains B. J. Kennedy, M.D., medical oncologist at the Fairview University Medical Center in Minneapolis, Minnesota, Regents' Professor of Medicine, Emeritus, and Masonic Professor of Oncology, Emeritus at the University of Minnesota.

Currently in the United States, most cancer cases (85 percent) are diagnosed in people over the age of 50. Kennedy was a pioneer in recognizing the implications of this fact. Shortly after he helped found the subspecialty of medical oncology in 1971, Kennedy began pushing for increased geriatric education for this newly formed division of internal medicine.

"Today, people are becoming increasingly aware that we're going to have a lot more older people, they are going to have a lot more cancer, and we're going to have to know how to treat them more effectively," Kennedy says.

Risk Rises over Time

In the United States, only 1 man in 69 develops cancer before the age of 40. That risk goes up to 1 in 12 for ages 40–59 and jumps to 1 in 3 for ages 60–79.

The statistics for women follow a similar pattern: only 1 woman in 52 develops some type of invasive cancer before the age of 40, but the figure rises to 1 in 11 for ages 40–59 and 1 in 5 for ages 60–79.

Cancer Risk and Age

This table lists the percentage of patients by age and type of cancer:

Cancer Type	Age in Years <40	40–49	50–64	>64
Prostate	<1	2	33	65
Breast	5	18	32	45
Lung	1	4	21	74
Colorectal	2	7	20	71
All Combined	5	10	26	59

Other physicians and organizations also recognized it was critical to put more resources into geriatric research. Their efforts culminated in the passage of the Research on Aging Act, resulting in the creation in 1974 of the National Institute on Aging, a branch of the National Institutes of Health that supports research and training related to the aging process and diseases, including cancer.

How Age and Cancer Are Related

The demographics clearly show that the incidence of most cancers increases with age. The reasons for this aren't as obvious.

William Ershler, M.D., director of the Institute for Advanced Studies in Aging and Geriatric Medicine in Washington, D.C., notes that cancer is more common in older people for a variety of reasons:

The Science behind Aging

Recent research has launched intriguing new theories that link the aging process and the development of cancer.

A body substance called *telomerase*, sometimes referred to as the "immortality enzyme," encourages cells to keep dividing indefinitely instead of dying with age. Some researchers have theorized that the study of telomerase could lead to important discoveries about the aging process and unlock secrets about cancer.

Another theory proposes that free radicals play a role both in aging and the development of cancer. A *free radical* is an atom or group of atoms that has at least one unpaired electron and is therefore unstable and highly reactive. In animal tissues, free radicals can damage cells and are believed to accelerate the progression of cancer and aging. Although *antioxidants* (substances such as vitamins C and E that protect the body's cells) "clean up" damage from free radicals, the process becomes less efficient as we age. Many scientists speculate that free radical damage is a primary culprit for age-related diseases and the symptoms of aging.

- **Time.** Ershler explains that it takes many years—even decades—for most cancers to develop. The types of cancers that occur most frequently in the elderly—colon, lung, prostate, and breast—are the kinds that take the longest to develop.

- **Diminished DNA repair mechanisms.** When potentially important fragments of DNA are damaged in a young and healthy person, the body's DNA repair mechanisms fix them. This capacity for DNA repair decreases with age.

- **Decline in immune function.** This theory suggests that as the body's immune system becomes less effective with age, people lose some of their ability to fight off malignancies.

Harvey Cohen, M.D., chief of geriatric medicine at Duke University Medical Center, says he doesn't think there is just one reason why cancer is more common in older people. It's likely that it is due to a combination of these factors—and possibly others that researchers haven't even uncovered yet.

The Color of Cancer: Race and Cancer Risk

Racial and ethnic minorities experience disproportionately greater suffering and compromised health from cancer compared to the U.S. population as a whole. Those most at risk for developing cancer are some of the fastest growing groups in our population.

American Indians and Alaska Natives

In the category of American Indians and Alaska Natives, there are over 560 federally recognized tribes and over 100 state recognized tribes, each of which has its own unique culture. Thus, there is great political, social, cultural, and spiritual diversity within American Indian and Alaska Native communities. Linguistic diversity also abounds: there are 217 native languages spoken today and most, if not all, indigenous languages do not include a word for "cancer."

Cancer rates that were previously reported to be lower in American Indians and Alaska Natives have been shown to be increasing in the past 20 years. In fact, American Indians and Alaska Natives now have some of the highest cancer mortality rates compared with other racial groups.

The type of cancer most often experienced within Native American communities varies according to geography. For example, among Alaska Natives, colon and lung cancers are diagnosed most frequently. Individuals from Northern Plains tribes have higher incidences of lung, cervical, breast, and prostate cancer, and southwestern tribe members are likelier to suffer from stomach and gallbladder cancer.

Asian Americans and Pacific-Islander Americans

Asians and Pacific Islanders (APIs) combined make up one of the fastest growing populations in the United States, increasing by more than 40 percent between 1990 and 2000.

The term Asian refers to people having familial origins in the Far East, Southeast Asia, or the Indian subcontinent. The Asian population includes many groups who differ in language, culture, and length of residence in the United States. Some Asian groups, like the Chinese and Japanese, have been in the United States for several generations. Other groups, such as the Hmong, Vietnamese, Laotians, and Cambodians, are comparatively recent immigrants.

According to the U.S. Census, Asian Americans account for 4.2 percent of the total U.S. population, or approximately 11.9 million people. The most populous Asian groups, in descending order, are the Chinese, Filipinos, and Asian Indians; combined, these three groups represent almost 60 percent of the Asian population in the United States.

According to the Asian American Network for Cancer Awareness, Research and Training, lung cancer is the leading cause of cancer death among Asian Americans and colorectal cancer is second. However, liver cancer is the third-leading cause of cancer death in Asian Americans, primarily due to high rates of exposure to and infection with the Hepatitis B virus in immigrant Asian populations (a leading cause of liver cancer), a critical difference between Asian Americans and other U.S. populations.

Cancer has been the number one killer of Asian-American women since 1980. Further, Asian-American females are the first U.S. population to experience cancer as the leading cause of death. Cervical cancer is a significant health problem in Vietnamese-American women, who are nearly five times as likely to develop and die from cervical cancer as white women. Vietnamese-American men have the highest rate of liver cancer in any racial and ethnic group in the United States, developing liver and bile duct cancer 11 times more often than white men. Korean-American men have the highest incidence of stomach cancer in the U.S., receiving this diagnosis five times more often than white men.

Susan Shinagawa's Story

Susan Shinagawa's doctor told her not to worry when she detected a lump in her breast 11 years ago. She was only 34 years old, he reassured her, too young to get breast cancer, and she had no family history of the disease. "Besides," he said, "Asian women don't get breast cancer."

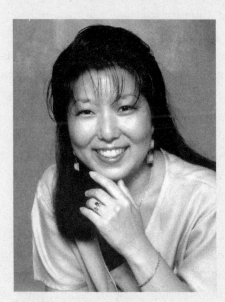

Susan Shinagawa

Luckily, she sought a second opinion and insisted on a biopsy of the lump. Shinagawa is now a cancer survivor and activist and has served as chair of the Intercultural Cancer Council, the nation's largest organization addressing cancer disparities in U.S. communities of color and poverty. She also cofounded the Asian & Pacific Islander National Cancer Survivors Network in 1998 and serves as community director for the Asian American Network for Cancer Awareness, Research and Training.

The *International Journal of Cancer* recently reported that the breast cancer incidence for Japanese-American women in Los Angeles has risen dramatically and is now nearly as high as, or has possibly even surpassed the incidence for white women.

Even in Japan, incidence rates are increasing. They more than doubled from 1960 to the late 1980s and are continuing to rise as the population adopts a more Western lifestyle.

Although there is conflicting data about what role diet plays in breast cancer, many known risk factors for the disease are associated with a Westernized lifestyle, like delaying childbirth beyond the age of 30, becoming overweight, not exercising enough, and drinking alcohol. Nonetheless, breast cancer rates for Japanese-American women are still significantly higher than those of Japanese women in Japan.

Pacific Islanders number just under 400,000—approximately 0.1 percent of the total U.S. population in 2000. This small group is comprised of more than 25 diverse subgroups with variations in historical backgrounds, languages, and cultural traditions. Among Pacific Islanders in the United States, Native Hawaiians are the largest group, followed by Samoans, Chamorros, Tongans, and Fijians. Seventy-five percent of Pacific Islanders live in California and Hawaii.

Inadequate data collection means there is very little reliable information about cancer in Pacific Islander populations. What we do know is chilling: Native Hawaiians have the highest cancer mortality rate of all racial and ethnic groups except African Americans. Residents of the Republic of the Marshall Islands (a former U.S. territory) have much higher cancer rates than residents of the United States, due to exposure to nuclear bomb testing and the dumping of nuclear waste on the Islands' atolls.

African Americans

African Americans constitute 12.7 percent of the total U.S. population. The African American community includes people from Nigeria, Ethiopia, South Africa, the West Indies, and other parts of the Caribbean.

African Americans have higher rates of lung, prostate, and colorectal cancers than other ethnic groups. A matter of particular concern is that African-American men have a 60 percent higher incidence of prostate cancer than white men.

African Americans are more likely to develop and die from cancer than persons of any other racial and ethnic group. African Americans are about one-third more likely to die of cancer than whites and more than twice as likely to die of cancer as Asians, Pacific Islanders, American Indians, and Hispanics. Although African Americans have experienced higher rates of cancer for many years, there is some good news: cancer deaths among African Americans have decreased substantially since 1991.

Breast Cancer Pathology:
Are the Differences Black and White?

Breast cancer affects different groups of American women in different ways. For example, African-American women are less likely to be diagnosed with breast cancer, but they are more likely to die from the disease once it is found. What accounts for these differences?

Social factors, such as diet, lifestyle, and unequal access to healthcare, may play a role. But there may also be *pathological*, or disease-related, differences in tumor characteristics between races. As an example, African-American women have a higher rate of premenopausal breast cancer than white women and are more than twice as likely to be diagnosed with specific types of tumors that are more aggressive and difficult to treat.

Researchers are still unsure of what accounts for these differences. After studying more than 90,000 women with breast cancer, researchers interested in ethnic differences concluded that "a combination of biological, genetic, environmental, and lifestyle differences across these populations are likely to account for these variations."

Lovell A. Jones, Ph.D., directs the Center for Research on Minority Health at the University of Texas, M.D. Anderson Cancer Center. A respected authority on race and cancer, Jones is interested in pinning down the reasons why the cancer mortality rate is higher for African Americans than for whites. Conventional wisdom suggests that such differences are a result of delayed access to treatment for African Americans, but Jones notes that such presumptions have very little scientific basis.

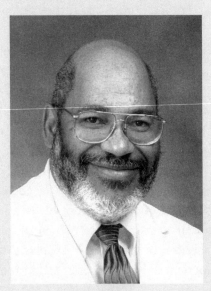

Lovell A. Jones, Ph.D.

The subject is controversial, and even experts disagree about the relative impact of genetics versus access to treatment. Jones asserts, "We have very little knowledge about the biology of the disease, and we have made a lot of assumptions based on data that was generated in terms of white females. That may not hold true for African-American women and other women of color."

One recent study suggests that access to treatment as a result of lower socioeconomic status may not be the only factor at play. The study, which took socioeconomic factors into account, demonstrated that race alone increased the mortality rate for African-American women about 20 percent compared to white women, suggesting that breast cancer behaves differently in African-American and white women, and that ethnicity is an independent predictor of a worse breast cancer outcome.

Caucasians

Caucasians account for approximately 75 percent of the U.S. population. The Caucasian (or white) population is made up of individuals with origins from any of the original peoples of Europe, the Middle East, or North Africa.

According to the U.S. Census, the white population grew at less than half the rate of the total population between 1990 and 2000.

The risk of skin cancer is about ten times higher for whites than for African Americans because of the protective effect of skin pigment. Whites with fair skin that freckles or burns easily are at especially high risk. Whites also have higher rates of testicular cancer, bladder cancer, and leukemia than other populations.

Hispanics

Hispanics are the fastest-growing population in the United States. According to the U.S. Census, the Hispanic population of the United States now outnumbers the non-Hispanic black population, with 13 percent of the population identifying themselves as Hispanic.

Hispanics are difficult to classify because they are a loosely defined ethnic group from many different countries and regions who share linguistic roots.

Most of the Hispanics, or Latinos, in the United States come from, in decreasing order, Mexico, Central or South America, Puerto Rico, and Cuba. Cancer occurrence varies across these groups because of regional, behavioral, and/or genetic differences.

In general, the cancer incidence rates among people of Hispanic origin are lower than among non-Hispanics. But while Hispanic women have lower rates of breast cancer incidence than either black or white women, Hispanic women have lower survival rates than whites. In addition, the incidence of stomach, liver, gallbladder, and cervical cancers is higher among Hispanics than the general population and is especially high among first-generation migrants to the United States.

Barriers to Reducing Cancer in Minority Populations

Ethnic and racial minority groups suffer a disproportionately high rate of cancer for many reasons, including language barriers, cultural differences, and the medical community's lack of knowledge about diverse populations.

The following charts show different races' screening rates for breast and cervical cancers—that is, how often people of various races and ethnicities are examined for these cancers although they have no symptoms:

Mammography and Race*

Race/Ethnicity	%[†]
White (non-Hispanic)	68
Black (non-Hispanic)	66
Hispanic	61
American Indian/Alaska Native	45
Asian/Pacific Islander	61

*These are 1998 statistics showing women 40 years and older in the United States who had a mammogram within the past two years.
†Percentages are age-adjusted to the 2000 U.S. standard population.

Pap Test and Race*

Race/Ethnicity	%[†]
White (non-Hispanic)	80
Black (non-Hispanic)	83
Hispanic	74
American Indian/Alaska Native	72
Asian/Pacific Islander	67

*These are 1998 statistics showing women 40 years and older in the United States who had a Pap test within the past three years.
†Percentages are age-adjusted to the 2000 U.S. standard population.

Source: National Health Interview Survey, 1998, National Center for Health Statistics, Centers for Disease Control and Prevention. American Cancer Society, Surveillance Research.

Language

Language barriers pose special problems to newly arriving immigrants. For example, Elmer Huerta, M.D., M.P.H., notes that many minorities such as Latinos do not have good access to the latest news about cancer prevention due to language barriers.

Huerta is the founder and director of the Cancer Preventorium at the Washington Hospital Center's Cancer Institute in Washington, D.C., which targets the Latino population. He hosts a nationally syndicated radio program called *Cuidando su Salud* (*Taking Care of Your Health*) to help break down language barriers and encourage Latinos to take good care of their health.

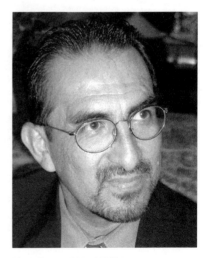

"Up to 60 percent of Latinos living in the United States were born outside of this country," says Huerta, a native of Peru. "They come here and they work two or three jobs, from early in the morning until night. They just forget about their bodies. I try to move them from inaction to action through education and screening."

Elmer Huerta, M.D., M.P.H.

Culture

When individuals immigrate to America from other countries, they may bring with them traditions and beliefs that clash with the prevailing medical practices in the United States.

Susan Shinagawa provides an example: "Cancer is a difficult subject in any culture, but especially among many Asians," she says. "A lot of it is cultural. You just don't talk about cancer or other problems." She adds, "You don't want to shame your family. There are a lot of fears and myths out there. Many Asians and Asian Americans believe cancer is contagious. Some Asians believe that you get cancer because you're being punished for something you—or one of your ancestors—did wrong. It's your karma and there's nothing you can do about it." It wasn't until eight years after her first primary breast cancer diagnosis that Shinagawa met more than a handful of Asian American breast cancer survivors, in large part, she believes, because of these and other cultural barriers.

"Culture doesn't cause cancer," says Stephen McPhee, M.D., a professor of medicine at the University of California in San Francisco and a cancer control researcher with the Vietnamese Community Health Promotion Project. "But," he adds, "cultural beliefs can contribute to the lack of prevention, as well as a lack of detection and treatment."

Inadequate Research

The process of compiling medical data for minority groups is enormously challenging, especially when the groups themselves are quite diverse. For example, there are a lot of cultural differences within the API population, says Shinagawa, making it difficult to generalize about larger populations.

Compiling reliable medical data is vital in helping health care providers target the specific needs of diverse populations. In some cases, however, cancer databases are rudimentary or nonexistent. For instance, with the exception of Native Hawaiians who reside in Hawaii, there is no systematic data collection on cancer incidence and mortality for Pacific Islanders.

According to the Intercultural Cancer Council, more comprehensive epidemiological research is needed to document accurately the scope of cancer in minority communities. Such research will help the medical community design more effective programs and treatment.

More Than Skin Deep: Economics and Cancer Risk

An estimated 33 million people live in poverty—just under 12 percent of the U.S. population. The main features of poverty that affect cancer detection, treatment, and survival of cancer include:

- unemployment

- inadequate education

- substandard housing

- chronic malnutrition

- diminished access to medical care

Individuals of all ethnic backgrounds who are poor experience higher cancer incidence, higher mortality rates, and poorer survival rates. Overall, the cancer survival rate of poor individuals is 10 to 15 percent lower than those of other Americans.

In addition to lower survival rates, poor people endure greater pain and suffering from cancer. They also have difficulty obtaining and using health care, effectively barring their access to quality cancer screening and treatment. Studies have shown that poor people tend not to seek care if they cannot pay for it, and that fatalism about cancer is prevalent among the poor because of an overwhelming sense of powerlessness. Finally, given their abject circumstances, the poorest Americans may focus only on day-to-day survival.

Lack of education is another reason—perhaps the central one— that cancer mortality rates are higher in poor populations. Cancer screening is less common among adults with low income and less education, as illustrated in the charts below. As an example, the difference in mammography screening for women who completed at least one year of college versus women who did not finish high school is 20 percent. The difference in Pap test screening between these levels of education is more than 15 percent. Increasing knowledge and creating access to affordable tests are important factors in eliminating the barriers to cancer screening.

Mammography and Education*

Education (years)	%[†]
11 or fewer	53
12	66
13 or more	73

* These are 1998 statistics for women 40 and older in the United States who had a mammogram within the past two years.
†Percentages are age-adjusted to the 2000 U.S. standard population.

Pap Test and Education*

Education (years)	%[††]
11 or fewer	69
12	78
13 or more	85

* These are 1998 statistics for women 40 and older in the United States who had a Pap test within the past three years.
†Percentages are age-adjusted to the 2000 U.S. standard population.
‡Women 25 years or older.

Source: National Health Interview Survey, 1998, National Center for Health Statistics, Centers for Disease Control and Prevention. American Cancer Society, Surveillance Research.

"Poverty drives certain negative events," says Freeman. "Poor people have substandard living conditions, less social support. They have less knowledge and are less educated. Poor people tend to have more of a risk-promoting lifestyle. They tend to have less access to health care, particularly to early preventive health care. You have to look at all those things."

The Double Whammy: When Minority Status and Poverty Overlap

In 2001, the poverty rate for whites was 7.8 percent, while poverty rates for racial and ethnic minorities were significantly higher: 24.5 percent for American Indians and Alaska Natives, 22.7 percent for Blacks, 21.4 percent for Hispanics, and 10.2 percent for Asians and Pacific Islanders.

Minority status and low socioeconomic status can overlap to create significant barriers for cancer prevention and control. Low income and less education—more common among some minority groups—can translate into diets higher in fat and lower in fruits and vegetables and more smoking, both known to increase risk of several cancers.

Leveling the Playing Field

All Americans—regardless of race or socioeconomic status—should have access to a health care system that provides cancer prevention, detection, and treatment services. The Intercultural Cancer Council has suggested the following policy principles to eliminate the unequal burden of cancer on racial and ethnic minorities and on the poor:

- Research must accurately record the scope of cancer in minority and medically underserved communities.

- Much higher priority must be given to research and control programs on cancers disproportionately affecting minorities and the medically underserved.

- Health materials must be culturally appropriate.

- Health care providers should be more sensitive and culturally competent.

- Minorities and culturally diverse individuals must have major roles in developing health policies and programs.

- Educational efforts should be enacted to counteract fatalism and overcome fears.

- Preventive health education and medical benefits must be provided in a variety of health care settings.

As cancer registries and epidemiological studies continue to add to researchers' knowledge about why and where cancer occurs, organizations like the National Cancer Institute, the Centers for Disease Control and Prevention, and the American Cancer Society continue to educate the public about screening and try to increase awareness about cancer, its risk factors, and its symptoms. As you have seen, much work remains to be done on the forefront of cancer control—especially within minority and medically underserved populations, who currently face some of the toughest obstacles obtaining quality health care.

In this chapter, we looked at how factors like age, race, and socioeconomic status affect our risk of developing cancer. In the next few chapters, we'll turn our attention to other variables that can affect our cancer risk—factors like genetics that we *can't* control, and factors like diet, physical activity, and tobacco use that we *can*.

CHAPTER 3

Why Does Cancer Develop?

KYLE RATTRAY WAS THREE AND A HALF YEARS OLD in 1986 when he fell from the front porch of his family's farmhouse in Sunnyside, Washington. Later that day, blood appeared in his urine. After several frustrating weeks of testing, a tumor was found on his right kidney and he was diagnosed with a rare kidney cancer that strikes children: *Wilms' tumor* (also called *nephroblastoma*). Like many children, Rattray was confused about cancer. "For the longest time I thought cancer was caused by a hard fall," he says.

Rattray underwent surgery to remove the diseased kidney and received months of chemotherapy. He lost his hair and he was nauseous, in pain, and terrified. Fortunately, the treatment was successful.

But over the years, the mystery of what caused his illness consumed Rattray, and he began devouring every book he could find on cancer. He soon became convinced that his destiny was to leave the family farm to become a physician. By the age of 16, he landed a

National Cancer Institute (NCI) research internship typically reserved for college students.

Today, Rattray is a 19-year-old student at the Massachusetts Institute of Technology, where he is assisting a team of scientists studying the genetic profile of Wilms' tumor.

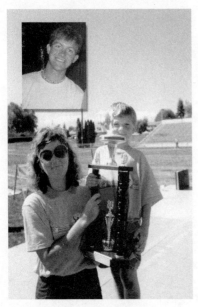

In the 16 years since Rattray was diagnosed with Wilms' tumor, major technological advances in the fields of molecular biology and *genetics* (the study of the inheritance of traits, variations, and disorders in organisms) have allowed knowledge about the cancer process to explode. Although genes were long suspected as culprits, only in recent decades have scientists been able to identify many of the genes directly involved in causing cancer.

Rattray, the once-frightened child who thought his cancer was caused by a fall, is now assisting biomedical researchers as they zero in on the genes connected with the disease that struck him. He spends hours doing the painstaking work of dissecting tiny mouse kidneys, transferring cell samples to slides, staining them with chemicals, and then looking for changes in the cells under a microscope. The work is often tedious but Rattray doesn't mind. "It's really exciting to me," he says.

Kyle Rattray at age 5, immediately following chemotherapy treatments for Wilms' tumor, accepting a spirit award at an American Cancer Society Relay for Life event.
Inset: Kyle Rattray at age 19.

What Is Cancer?

Normal body cells grow, divide, and die in an orderly fashion. Normal cells typically divide more rapidly in a person's early years, slowing down when the person becomes an adult. At that point, cells in most parts of the body divide only to replace worn-out or dying cells and to repair injuries.

Cancer cells don't know when to stop growing and dividing. Instead of dying after a certain number of replications, they continue to form new abnormal cells. These abnormal cells don't follow the rules of normal cells either, continuing to divide into increasingly abnormal cells, destroying tissues around them, and spreading through the body.

Robert Weinberg writes in his book *One Renegade Cell: How Cancer Begins*, "The cancer cell is a renegade. Unlike their normal counterparts, cancer cells disregard the needs of the community of cells around them. Cancer cells are only interested in their own pro-liferative advantage. They are selfish and very unsociable. Most important, unlike normal cells, they have learned to grow without any prompting from the community of cells around them."

"Cancer cells become immortal," adds Len Lichtenfeld, M.D., medical editor for the American Cancer Society (ACS). "They keep reproducing and all their different cellular mechanisms become altered."

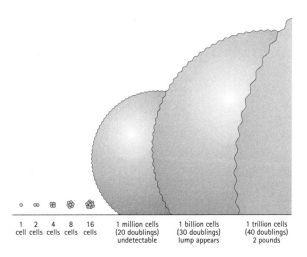

| 1 cell | 2 cells | 4 cells | 8 cells | 16 cells | 1 million cells (20 doublings) undetectable | 1 billion cells (30 doublings) lump appears | 1 trillion cells (40 doublings) 2 pounds |

Cancer cells grow and divide unchecked.

This process of spreading, called *metastasis*, occurs when the cancer cells get into the bloodstream or lymph vessels and travel to other parts of the body. Cancer is generally named after the body tissue where it began. For example, even when cells from a cancer in the breast spread to the liver, the cancer is still called breast cancer, not liver cancer.

"Your normal skin cells don't go to your eyes and your foot cells don't go to your head, but cancer cells have the ability to break off, enter the bloodstream, and go to another part of the body," explains Lichtenfeld.

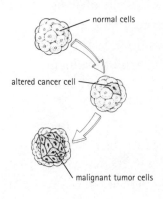

normal cells

altered cancer cell

malignant tumor cells

How a tumor begins.

Over time, the cells may begin to grow and replace normal tissue, forming tumors. Tumors are abnormal growths of cells or tissues that can be *malignant* (cancerous) or *benign* (noncancerous). Benign tumors do not spread to other parts of the body and are usually not life threatening. Cancer often forms as a solid tumor, but some cancers, like leukemia, do not form tumors. These cancer cells involve the blood and blood-forming organs and circulate through other tissues, where they grow.

DNA and the Gene Scene

Cancer cells develop because of damage to deoxyribonucleic acid, or DNA, a substance in every cell that directs the growth, division, and other functions of cells. Most of the time when DNA becomes damaged, the cell dies or is able to repair the damage. But in cancer cells, some of the damaged DNA is not repaired.

DNA determines hair color, eye color, and any inherited trait—including the susceptibility to some diseases. People inherit DNA from their parents. People can inherit damaged DNA, thus inheriting a greater risk of cancer. Many times, though, a person's DNA becomes damaged during the course of his or her lifetime by exposure to something in the environment, like smoking. (We'll talk more about environmental and lifestyle factors that cause cancer in chapters 5, 6, and 7.)

Chromosomes are threadlike bodies in the nucleus of a cell that carry the chemical "instructions" for reproduction of the cell. They consist of strands of DNA wrapped in a double helix around a core of proteins. Each species of plant or animal has a characteristic number of chromosomes; for example, humans have 46 chromosomes.

Chromosomes carry genes. Genes are segments of DNA. Genes tell the cell to do a specific task, usually to make a particular protein. Each human cell has about 100,000 genes; each gene makes a protein with a unique job. Certain proteins, for example, help the cell divide into two cells and others prevent the cell from dividing too often.

Not all genes "run" continuously. A cell uses its genes selectively. It activates, or "turns on," the genes it needs at the right moment. Some genes stay active all the time to produce proteins needed for basic cell functions.

Genes that help a cell grow and divide normally are called *proto-oncogenes*. When these genes mutate (become altered or changed), they can become *onco-genes*, which allow cells to divide too quickly and become cancer cells. It may be helpful to think of a cell as a car. For it to work properly, there needs to a way to control how fast it goes. A proto-

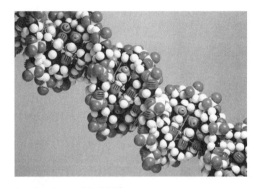

A molecular model of DNA.

oncogene normally functions in a way that is similar to a gas pedal—it helps the cell grow and divide. An oncogene could be compared to a gas pedal that is stuck down, which causes the cell to divide out of control. Researchers are studying ways to try to switch off oncogenes to stop cancer growth.

A *tumor suppressor gene* is like the brake pedal on a car; just as a brake keeps a car from going too fast, a tumor suppressor gene keeps the cell from dividing too quickly. Tumor suppressor genes also tell cells when to repair damaged DNA and when to die (a normal process called *apoptosis*, or programmed cell death). When tumor suppressor genes are mutated or turned off—that is, when the brakes fail, they allow cells to divide too fast, allowing cancer cells to develop. Abnormalities in tumor suppressor genes can be inherited, or they can be acquired during a person's life.

Changing Lives

Oncogenes and tumor suppressor genes have a lot to offer researchers as targets for cancer therapies. Current clinical trials of drugs that affect these genes will likely lead to better treatments for many types of cancer. Discoveries about oncogenes and tumor suppressor genes have already helped researchers improve the quality of life and prolong the lives of some people with cancer. Here are just a couple of examples:

Gleevec

The introduction of the new drug *Gleevec* (generic name imatinib mesylate; another trade name is STI571) has completely changed how doctors treat people with *chronic myelogenous leukemia (CML)*. The development of CML seems to be driven by an abnormal molecule, the *bcr-abl* protein (a product of the *bcr-abl* oncogene). The Gleevec pill inhibits this protein so well that almost all patients respond to the drug. In fact, well over 90 percent of patients have a complete *remission* (disease-free period) of their leukemia.

Until Gleevec, high-dose chemotherapy and total body irradiation followed by stem cell transplantation were the only known treatments for CML. But the side effects of stem cell transplantation are serious and can be fatal. Gleevec's side effects are much less extensive. For people with CML, Gleevec is a dream come true.

Gleevec has recently been approved for treatment of gastro-intestinal stromal tumor, and is now being studied for use with other cancers as well.

Herceptin

Herceptin (generic name trastuzumab) is a drug that works by preventing the *HER2/neu* protein (another oncogene product) from promoting excessive growth of cancer cells. Herceptin attaches to HER2/neu, which is found in high numbers on the surface of many breast cancer cells. Herceptin can stop the HER2/neu protein from making breast cancer cells grow.

Herceptin can shrink some breast cancer metastases that return after chemotherapy or continue to grow during chemotherapy. Used alone or together with chemotherapy drugs, Herceptin can shrink some breast cancers that have high levels of HER2/neu and help women who have these cancers live longer. In comparison with chemotherapy drugs, the side effects of Herceptin are relatively mild. Studies are currently underway to see if it will be useful in treating people with other cancers.

When a Good Cell Turns Bad: How Cancer Develops

Cancer doesn't happen overnight. Its development is a lengthy process that starts when genes are damaged. A person can inherit damaged DNA, or chemicals and toxins in the environment can damage DNA.

The process that changes normal cells into cancer is called *carcinogenesis*. The chemicals and other exposures that cause these changes and increase the risk of cancer are called carcinogens. Chemicals in tobacco smoke, viruses like the human papillomavirus (HPV), radiation from radiotherapy machines, and ultraviolet rays from the sun are carcinogens. Even though researchers have pinpointed various stages in the development of some cancers, such as colon cancer, much about carcinogenesis remains a mystery.

In recent decades, molecular biology research has provided more answers about carcinogenesis. Childhood cancers such as Wilms' tumor are believed to be the result of only a few cellular mutations and do not require much time to develop. But many of the cancers that occur in adulthood require a whole series of cellular alterations and can take years or even decades to grow into a detectable tumor.

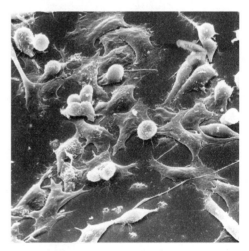

A picture of Wilms' tumor magnified 130 times, taken with a scanning electron microscope. Image courtesy of Dr. Timothy Triche and the National Cancer Institute.

"The process is so complex," says Herman Kattlove, M.D., medical editor for the ACS. "If you look at the charts of cancer pathways and how cancer forms, there are hundreds of steps along the way."

Our cells are constantly subjected to influences that might cause them to divide incorrectly, but the body has an amazing ability to correct itself. It is not easy to get cancer. It takes years, Kattlove explains, which means you have years to do something about it.

Step-by-Step: Stages of Cancer Development

Damage to a cell's DNA is called a mutation. Mutations are common, occurring a million or more times in the body each day. Almost all of these mutations are repaired, and those that cannot be repaired are usually eliminated when the mutated cell dies. But sometimes a mutation escapes repair. In that case, when the cell divides, the mutation is passed on to the next generation of cells. As cells continue to divide, the mutation may continue to be passed on. If it is a harmless mutation, it may never be noticed. But if the mutation happens to lead to uncontrolled cell growth, it may result in cancer.

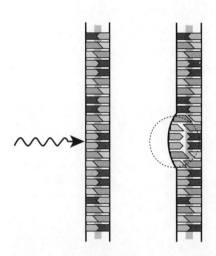

During the first few decades of the twentieth century, scientists discovered that some chemicals could trigger cellular changes that could eventually develop into cancer. These chemicals were called *initiators*, and it later became clear that they acted on the cell's genetic material, DNA. Once an initiator had made the initial changes in a cell, other chemicals

Damage to a cell's DNA is called a mutation. Some cell mutations are harmless. Others may lead to cancer. Image adapted from Andrew Hutchins, ©1997–2000.

called *promoters* would prompt further changes that would lead the cell to become cancerous. From these observations, scientists concluded that cancer developed in steps—the concept known as *multistage carcinogenesis*.

This process requires several different events, which take place over time, sometimes many years. This explains why there is a delay, or *latency period*, between exposure to a carcinogen and the development of cancer. Researchers believe this period corresponds to the stages of *initiation, promotion,* and *progression.*

Initiation: Carcinogenesis begins when one or more oncogenes or tumor suppressor genes are mutated. They then alter a cell's normal programming, causing it to reproduce abnormal versions of itself. This initial damage to one of these critical genes can be inherited, or it can be acquired over time by exposures to cancer-causing influences known as initiators.

Promotion: Some carcinogens do not cause DNA damage but drive altered cells to grow, stepping up the process of carcinogenesis. These carcinogens, known as promoters, can occur naturally in the body. Some examples are bile acids, estrogens, and androgens. Some substances, including many of the chemicals in tobacco, act as both initiators and promoters.

Tumor Progression: In its early stages, a cancer may lack the ability to metastasize, or spread. But as the cancer cells grow and become more aggressive, they may:

- break through the walls of blood vessels and move to other organs of the body, where they attach themselves and grow;

- form new blood vessels (a process known as *angiogenesis*) and divert nourishment to themselves more effectively;

- evade the body's immune system by camouflaging themselves or producing fewer *antigens* (foreign substances that signal the body's immune system to destroy them) on their surfaces, thus escaping detection and destruction.

How Colon Cancer Develops

Colon cancer typically develops slowly. Researchers believe it can take as long as 20 years for the initial changes in the cells that line the intestine to progress into a malignancy. This means that relatively small changes in the cells of the large intestine can be detected before they develop into cancer. A *colonoscope*, an optic tube inserted into the rectum, enables a doctor to check the colon for *polyps* (projectile growths of tissue into the center of the colon or rectum).

Most colorectal cancers begin as a polyp, also known as *adenoma*. Over many years these can slowly change into cancer. Some types of polyps, for example, inflammatory polyps, are not precancerous. But having *adenomatous polyps*, or small benign tumors, increases your risk of developing cancer, especially if you have many polyps or if they are large.

Once a polyp becomes cancerous, it may metastasize by penetrating the lining of the intestine and moving into other parts of the body, usually the nearby lymph nodes and the liver.

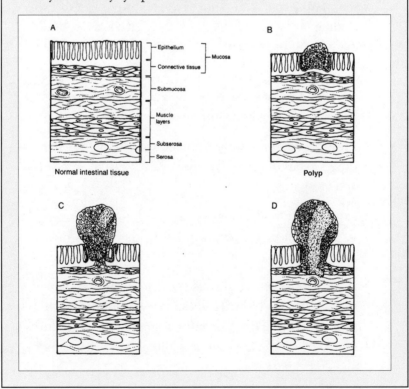

Sometimes Cancer Is a Family Affair

Recent breakthroughs in genetics, such as the mapping of the complete human genome (the approximately 30,000 genes in the human body), have changed the way scientists study complex diseases like cancer.

"It completely transforms how we do things in my lab," says Barbara Lynn Weber, M.D., of the University of Pennsylvania Cancer Center. "Before, it was like looking into a box with a billion different puzzle pieces in it. Now, we are looking at the puzzle all put together."

Our growing knowledge of the human genome has allowed scientists to identify and study gene mutations or abnormalities that are passed down through families.

The recent media hype about these inherited mutations has contributed to a common misconception—that cancer is largely an inherited disease. If you are like most people, you are not destined to develop breast cancer just because your mother did or prostate cancer for the simple reason that your Uncle Joe had it. In fact, up to 70 percent of serious diseases can be prevented or delayed by making healthy lifestyle choices. Only a small percentage of fatal cancers are related to inherited gene mutations.

"Many people don't understand the difference between inheriting damaged genes and inheriting good genes that become damaged during their lifetimes," says Robert Weinberg, Ph.D., a member of the Whitehead Institute for Biomedical Research in Cambridge, Massachusetts. "Ninety percent of cancer is caused by genes that are damaged after you leave the womb." (In chapters 5, 6, and 7, we discuss environmental factors and lifestyle choices that affect our cancer risk.)

DNA contains the genetic code that gives orders to all human cells. Prior to discoveries about the nature of DNA, scientists knew only that sometimes cancer seemed to run in families. But today, armed with increased understandings of DNA and the human genome, scientists are identifying specific genes that, when inherited, can lead to cancer.

Linking Genetics and Cancer: Li-Fraumeni Syndrome

In the late 1960s, Frederick Li, M.D., was fresh from medical school and getting advanced training as a researcher in the epidemiology branch of the NCI.

During rounds with the clinicians, he was introduced to a puzzling case: a one-year-old boy had been diagnosed with a sarcoma, a rare type of cancer, in his bicep. The boy's cousin, another one year old, had been diagnosed with a sarcoma in his deltoid muscle. "To have two children in a family with a rare cancer is like lightning striking twice in the same spot," Li says. "They were extraordinary."

Their case became even more intriguing when Li learned the history of their immediate family. One of the boys' fathers died of leukemia at the age of 25 and the other one's mother had breast cancer. Their distant relatives also had a high rate of cancer diagnosed at relatively young ages, including a third sarcoma. Some of the cancer-stricken relatives lived hundreds of miles away from each other, making an environmental factor highly unlikely.

It was known by that time that colon cancer tended to track in some families and breast cancer tended to track in others. What made this family's situation extraordinary was that the family's cancers were not of the same type and that family members were all quite young when they were diagnosed. "There obviously was something going on," says Li, currently a professor of clinical cancer epidemiology at Harvard School of Public Health and professor of medicine at Harvard University. "But if you looked at the published information at the time, there was not that much of a clue about what it could be."

The family was devastated, but they cooperated fully when Li began investigating their medical histories. The most he could offer them was hope for an explanation of what was happening to them, not a cure.

"The thing that impressed me was the tremendous courage they had," Li recalls. "It was very touching. They wanted to help with the research even though they were suffering. That's always been an inspiration to me."

Robert Miller, M.D., chief of the NCI epidemiology branch, and Joseph Fraumeni, M.D., section head of the branch, wanted Li to dig further. They sent him around the country to children's hospitals to see if he could find families with similar histories.

Li spent months in hospital record departments, looking through records of children with sarcoma. He eventually identified four families that each had two children diagnosed with soft-tissue sarcomas. The parents, grandparents, and other relatives of these children had a high frequency of cancers diagnosed at relatively young ages, including carcinomas of the breast, brain tumors, acute leukemia, and other cancers.

Li's findings showed that an inherited factor was the most likely explanation in what was to become known as *Li-Fraumeni syndrome*. People with this syndrome have a higher risk for developing a number of cancers, including soft-tissue and bone sarcomas, brain tumors, breast cancer, adrenal gland cancer, and leukemia. Although the syndrome is exceedingly rare, its identification was one in a series of important steps linking genetics to cancer.

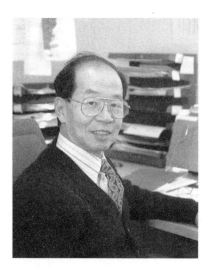

Frederick Li, M.D.

A Deeper Link: The "Two-Hit" Theory

As technology became more sophisticated, scientists were able dig even deeper into the connection between genes and cancer.

While studying *retinoblastoma*, a rare childhood eye tumor, Alfred G. Knudson Jr., M.D., Ph.D., developed a genetic model to explain how mutations in tumor suppressor genes play a role in the development of cancer. He showed that the loss of tumor suppressor gene function is involved in the development of both sporadic (not inherited) and hereditary cancers.

He observed that children in some families develop retinoblastoma at an early age, usually in both eyes, while children from families with no history of retinoblastoma tend to develop it later and only in one eye. In 1971, he suggested that this cancer resulted from two different genetic mutations, now called the "two-hit theory."

For example, in cases of retinoblastoma tumors, two genetic events, or "hits," affect the two normal copies of the tumor suppressor gene *RB*. In sporadic retinoblastoma tumors, both mutations occur in the retinal cells spontaneously, or as a result of environmental influences. In contrast, individuals who develop the hereditary form of retinoblastoma inherit the first defective copy of the *RB* gene from an affected parent, followed by the loss of the function of the second gene at some point after birth through a spontaneous mutation. Knudson's discovery of the *RB* gene as a tumor suppressor gene continues to serve as a model for other studies of genetic susceptibility to cancer.

The Guardian of the Genome: *p53*

In 1979, scientists discovered a gene they named *p53*. It was originally thought to be an oncogene that aided cells in dividing. But in 1989, Bert Vogelstein and his colleagues showed that *p53* is actually a tumor suppressor gene that, when mutated, allows cancer to form.

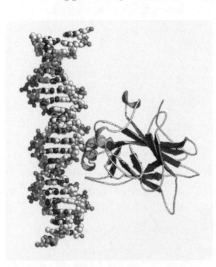

Normally, *p53* stops cell division when it detects damage to the DNA or forces the cell to die. But when there are defects in the gene, it loses its protective function. Studies show that defects in *p53* play a role in more than half of the cancers that occur in humans, including colon, breast, lung, bladder, brain, and liver cancer, and leukemia. Consequently, *p53* has been called the "guardian of the genome" and is the most widely studied gene in cancer research.

The tumor-suppressing *p53* protein can bind to target sequences on DNA to activate genes that prevent cell growth. Image courtesy of *The BioInformer*, European Bioinformatics Institute.

In 1990, Li and his colleagues made another important discovery. After decades of research on blood samples provided by families with similar clusters of cancer in children and young adults, Li and his colleagues discovered a common link among all the family members with Li-Fraumeni syndrome: inborn mutations in the *p53* gene. This established that the mutation of this gene could be inherited, if only rarely.

Today, approximately 30 tumor suppressor genes in addition to *p53* have been unmasked, including *APC*, and *BRCA1* and *BRCA2*. *APC* mutations are linked to *familial polyposis*, a condition that causes colon polyps to develop. These polyps can eventually become cancerous. Mutations in the *BRCA1* and *BRCA2* genes are associated with breast cancer.

The Breast Cancer Genes

Many centuries ago, physicians in ancient Rome noticed that breast cancer occurred more frequently in some families. But it was not until the 1990s that the *BRCA1* and *BRCA2* genes and their links to breast cancer were identified.

Weighing the Risks

- A woman with a *BRCA1* mutation is believed to have a 50 to 85 percent lifetime risk of developing breast cancer, compared with the average woman's risk of about 13 percent. *BRCA2* mutation carriers are thought to have a 40 to 80 percent risk of developing breast cancer.

- *BRCA1* and *BRCA2* mutations are also linked to cancers of the ovaries, prostate, and pancreas and to several other types of cancer, although the associated risk is not nearly as high as for breast cancer.

- Inherited gene mutations account for only about 5 percent of breast cancer cases overall. They are associated with an estimated 10 to 20 percent of breast cancer cases in younger women.

BRCA1 and *BRCA2* are often called the breast cancer genes—a bit of a misnomer, because the genes themselves do not cause cancer. *BRCA1* and *BRCA2* are actually tumor suppressor genes, which, under normal circumstances, help prevent cancer by making proteins that keep cells from growing abnormally. When *BRCA1* and *BRCA2* are mutated, tumor suppression no longer functions and cancer is more likely to develop.

Mutations in the normal *BRCA1* and *BRCA2* genes can be passed down through families, substantially raising the risk for breast cancer in those who inherit these mutations.

To Test or Not to Test?

As scientists unravel the mystery of DNA, they continue to identify genes that play a critical role in cancer. In some cases, scientists can identify people at high risk for developing cancer by testing for mutations in inherited genes. But *genetic testing* is a complicated business, and the decision to test or not to test is equally complex.

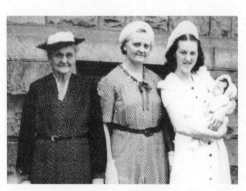

Four generations of women in a family. Image courtesy of the National Cancer Institute.

Genetic testing is conducted to see if a person has a certain gene mutation known to increase the risk for a specific disease (such as cancer), or to confirm a suspected mutation in an individual or family. Genetic testing is not recommended for everyone but is useful for people with specific types of family disease histories.

If you are concerned about your family history or other cancer risk factors, you may want to consider genetic testing. Doctors will sometimes recommend that a patient undergo genetic testing if there is a strong family history of a disease. This may include having more than two first-degree relatives (mother, father, sister, brother) with cancer, family members who developed cancer at a young age, relatives with rare cancers, or a known genetic mutation in your family.

Barbara Lynn Weber, M.D., is one of the many researchers who worked on isolating and mapping the *BRCA1* and *BRCA2* genes. Today she is a professor of medicine and genetics and director of the breast cancer program at the University of Pennsylvania Cancer Center in Philadelphia. She implemented the center's Breast Cancer Risk Evaluation Program, designed to provide risk assessment and counseling services to women, especially those with a family history of the disease.

Weber says that most individuals do not need testing. However, she recommends that anyone with a family history of breast cancer see a specialist for *genetic counseling*. Although Weber tends to encourage people to get tested if it seems at all likely that they carry a gene mutation, she says that in the end deciding whether to get tested is a personal decision.

Genetic Counseling

Genetic counseling takes place prior to genetic testing. The philosophy of genetic counseling is to present information in an unbiased or neutral fashion to allow individuals considering genetic testing to make their own decisions.

Genetic counselors have specialized training to help individuals understand how families inherit cancers and how genes are transmitted, as well as the types of cancer seen in the family and the individual's estimated risk. Counselors discuss benefits, risks, costs, and limitations of testing, and help individuals decide who in the family should be tested.

They also educate those considering genetic testing about the testing process, and help individuals and their families to cope with fears about test results, the potential for discrimination, and the risk of disease for children.

Weber notes that while many people are really scared of testing, "it can be extremely useful. It can help them to know their risk and take the appropriate preventive steps."

The Overlooked Branches of the Family Tree

If your sister, your mother, her mother, and all of your aunts are cancer free, does this mean that you have a family history free and clear of breast cancer? Not necessarily. Many women overlook their father's side of the family, which plays an equal role in determining the likelihood of inheriting a *BRCA1* or *BRCA2* gene mutation.

At the same time, people may overestimate their risk of cancer because they think it "runs in the family." What they neglect to do is look further into the branches of the family tree to understand the specific types and causes of cancer in their family. For example, Paul's grandfather had melanoma and his father developed lung cancer. He is immobilized with fear because he thinks he is also going to develop cancer. However, unlike breast and ovarian cancer, which have genetic links, there are no known genetic links between melanoma and lung cancer. If Paul looked a little deeper, he would begin to see the environmental links in his family instead. It turns out that his grandfather had red hair, light skin, and worked outdoors, and his father smoked two packs of cigarettes a day. So, Paul's risk of cancer probably has little to do with biology and a lot to do with lifestyle choices.

What If Testing Shows an Increased Risk of Developing Cancer?

When an individual decides to undergo genetic testing, specific laboratory tests are done to look at the genetic area of interest. This usually involves drawing blood or tissue samples from a tumor, skin, or fetus.

If the laboratory test result is positive (or inconclusive), the priority is to manage the risk through early detection testing, preventive surgery, or chemoprevention.

Early detection tests may be required more frequently if you have a positive test result. For example, a woman with a genetic mutation for breast cancer may need to undergo more frequent mammography exams to look for early signs of the cancer.

Preventive surgery (also called *prophylactic* surgery) is another option in some cases. A woman at high risk for developing ovarian cancer may decide to have her ovaries removed, for example.

Chemoprevention is the use of chemical agents to reverse, suppress, or prevent cells from developing into cancer. Several medicines are being studied to help prevent cancer from developing in high-risk patients.

What Are the Benefits of Testing?

For a person at risk for a specific cancer, a negative result on a genetic test may help reduce worry. Similarly, a positive result can help make important decisions about the future and may lead to finding disease earlier.

In addition, individual genetic testing can have wider implications. The ultimate goal of genetic testing research is to develop better methods of early detection, risk reduction, and disease prevention. The more information scientists can collect about cancer through genetic testing, the more able they will be to develop cancer treatments—and one day, cancer cures.

What Are the Issues Surrounding Testing?

Despite the potential benefits from the information we've learned about genes and their functions, serious concerns about medical, scientific, ethical, legal, and social issues have been raised because of the development and use of genetic tests.

In 1998, Donna Shalala, Department of Health and Human Services Secretary, convened the Secretary's Advisory Committee of Genetic Testing (SACGT). In March 2000, SACGT presented its preliminary recommendations on these issues:

- The Food and Drug Administration (FDA) should be involved in a timely and cost effective review of all new genetic tests.

- Federal legislation should prevent discrimination in employment and health insurance based on genetic information. Privacy of genetic information in medical records should be protected by legislation.

- Laboratories should ensure the quality of tests and share information about the clinical effectiveness and use of genetic tests. Confidentiality of testing results must be a priority in the process of data collection efforts.

The government also established the Ethical, Legal, and Social Implications (ELSI) Program to examine issues related to privacy, professional and public education, and ethical issues.

Why Should I Be Cautious About Testing?

A person considering genetic testing should carefully consider the following issues before being tested:

Limited answers

- Genetic tests can tell what *might* happen, but not what *will* happen. A positive test result does not necessarily mean a disease will occur. A negative result does not mean you have no risk.

- A test may be flawed.

- Test results may be misinterpreted.

Psychological impact

- Learning that you have or might develop a serious disease is frightening, especially if you have family members that have already died of the disease in question.

- Testing can strain family relationships. Family members who learn that they have a gene or have passed a gene on to their children may experience guilt and anger.

- Testing and waiting for results can produce stress and anxiety. (However, studies suggest that individuals at higher risk for a specific cancer who choose not to get tested or who receive unclear results are more likely to become depressed than individuals who receive an informative result, positive or negative.)

Privacy issues and discrimination

- Health Insurance: Over 20 percent of people with a genetic disorder report that they or a family member have been refused health insurance on the basis of their genetic profile.

- Employment: Eighty-five percent of Americans are afraid employers might have access to and use their genetic information to discriminate against them when making hiring or promotion decisions.

- Adoption: Some people are concerned that adoption efforts could be stopped based on sensitive genetic information.

Tools for Life

Just a generation ago, researchers suspected that cancer was related to DNA, but they had no idea how cancer really worked. Scientists have learned a lot about the nature and the course of cancer in recent years. In fact, their understanding of the molecular biology of cancers has exploded in just the past two decades. The ability to grow tumor cells *in vitro* (in test tubes) and to study the way they change and the factors that affect their growth has given scientists enormous insights into the basic mechanisms of cancer.

With the tools to identify specific genes involved in the cancer process, scientists have unlocked the door to help us understand more about what causes cancer and what doesn't. This has made all the difference to the many people whose cancers can be treated with molecularly targeted therapies.

"Since the 1960s and 1970s, when we started to gain a lot of ground in understanding what causes various cancers, we have built up quite a bit of knowledge," says Joseph Fraumeni, Jr., M.D., director of cancer epidemiology and genetics at NCI in Bethesda, Maryland. "Now we are at the point where molecular biology and molecular genetics are going to help us understand much of the rest of the picture."

CHAPTER 4

Making Sense of Scientific Studies

T HERE ARE OVER 100 MILLION CELLULAR PHONE USERS in the United States. Each year in this country, brain cancer occurs at a rate of about six new cases per 100,000 people. Is there a connection? Experts say probably not, but the public tends to focus on the miniscule "what if" rather than the preponderance of scientific evidence. Sensational stories featured in the media help fuel this attitude.

In 1993, David Reynard appeared on a national television talk show claiming that his pregnant wife developed (and later died from) a brain tumor from using her cellular phone. A grieving Reynard described how the brain tumor grew in the spot next to where the antenna was when his wife used her cell phone.

The program also featured a member of the committee of experts that spent years reviewing the scientific studies of radiofrequency energy and set the safety standards for cellular phones. The dry, scientific data he outlined was difficult to comprehend, and not very compelling. But the tragedy of a doomed young mother-to-be was clear enough.

Even though Reynard's lawsuit was later dismissed for lack of evidence, and a growing body of scientific evidence showed no consistent association between cellular phone use and brain cancer, almost a decade later, the same national talk show tackled the topic again, asking "Do cellular phones cause cancer?"

This time, Chris Newman, M.D., a neurologist, declared that his nine-year history of cell phone use was responsible for his brain cancer. He filed an $800 million lawsuit against his cell phone's maker and other cellular phone companies.

Again, a battery of experts debunked the claims of a connection between cancer and cellular phone use, including John Moulder, Ph.D., a cancer researcher and professor of radiation oncology at the Medical College of Wisconsin, who says, "The evidence that's out there now—and there's a lot of it—does not suggest any link."

Director of the Food and Drug Administration's (FDA) Center for Devices and Radiological Health, David Feigal M.D., M.P.H., concurs, "At this time there is no reason to conclude that there are health risks posed by cell phones to consumers." The FDA continues to look into the matter, though. The agency—with funding from the cell phone industry—is planning new studies. However, those results are not due for several years.

Even Moulder admits the limitations of science and the challenge of proving a negative correlation: "If you want a definitive answer— and definitive means absolute assurance of absolute safety—I'm afraid you're never going to get it because we just can't do it." However, he reasserts, "the current evidence does not indicate there's any problem, and there's a lot of research out there."

(For more information on cell phones and cancer risk, see pages 102–104).

Anecdotal Versus Scientific Evidence

Personal anecdotes hold tremendous power over the imagination. Journalists often use them to add drama and color to their reports and to draw people into the subject at hand. But anecdotes usually have little to do with scientific proof—even though they often overshadow it. Powerful testimonials about health disasters create lingering fears and suspicions for many of us. Meanwhile researchers rigorously and repeatedly run experiments, trying to get to the truth by stripping away study results that are not an example of cause and effect, but of chance occurrences.

Scientific research takes time. Studies often need to be repeated and confirmed. The answers they provide often aren't headline grabbing and are at times mundane. And many times they aren't clear-cut. Understandably, people want answers, and sometimes it's hard to accept that researchers just don't have them—at least not yet.

It may take decades to settle the debate scientifically. Meanwhile, the media will report the results of each study—and lawsuit—to satisfy the public's immediate need for information.

John Boice, Sc.D., scientific director of the International Epidemiology Institute in Rockville, Maryland, offers this advice to people concerned about the possible health effects of any new technology or product: "Don't look for the latest study—look for consistency across studies." Health recommendations from organizations like the American Cancer Society (ACS) are not based solely on one study because each study contributes only a piece to the larger puzzle.

Headline Horrors

One morning in 1981, as coffee drinkers across America poured their first cups of java and opened up their daily newspapers, they were confronted with this news: A study showed that coffee drinking might account for cases of pancreatic cancer, one of the deadliest forms of cancer. Follow-up studies would fail to confirm any link between coffee drinking and pancreatic cancer. It became evident that the first study had likely been a statistical fluke.

In 1989, *Alar* (daminozide) hit the headlines. The growth regulator used by apple farmers went through rigorous FDA testing before it was approved for use in the 1960s. But later tests found that mice fed extremely high doses of Alar developed tumors. A national television news program reported that Alar might be causing childhood cancers, and terrified parents stopped putting apples in their children's lunchboxes. Millions of dollars worth of apples were dumped. Later studies showed that Alar is probably less toxic than originally believed. A panel of members from the United Nations World Health Organization (WHO) and the Food and Agriculture Organization (FAO) ruled that trace amounts of Alar were acceptable in agricultural products. But in the United States, the furor about Alar had tipped over the apple cart.

The molecular structure of Alar, the trade name for a chemical sprayed on plants to retard growth and increase storage life. Apple image courtesy of Renee Comet and the National Cancer Institute. Molecular structure of Alar courtesy of the National Toxicology Program.

These are just a few of the dozens of examples of chemicals and products that loom large in the news for a while as a possible cancer risk and then often evaporate from the headlines and the public consciousness.

We've come a long way from just 50 years ago when the word "cancer" was commonly considered unmentionable in polite company. Today, cancer is a popular topic with the media, routinely cropping up in newspapers, and on TV and radio reports. Countless Internet sites—many of which have hidden agendas—are further complicating matters.

Science is becoming an increasing part of our everyday lives. Newspapers now publish entire science and health sections. People are eager to understand this complex information because they know it affects them. Everyday people want to know how their bodies work, and it's important to have the information explained in a clear way.

Unfortunately, scientific subtleties are often lost when journalists, attempting to meet daily deadlines, streamline complicated information into easily digestible and sensational headlines and stories. Sometimes the public gets an exaggerated message about a possible cancer risk without getting the necessary background information to help them make sense of it.

Reading Between the (Head) Lines

In his book *A Mathematician Reads the Newspaper*, John Allen Paulos writes:

> Consider a headline that invites us to infer a causal connection: *"Bottled Water Linked to Healthier Babies."* Without further evidence, this invitation should be refused, since affluent parents are more likely both to drink bottled water and to have healthy children; they have the stability and wherewithal to offer good food, clothing, shelter, and amenities. Families that own cappuccino makers are more likely to have healthy babies for the same reason.

Paulos warns of leaping to such conclusions. "Making a practice of questioning correlations when reading about 'links' between this practice and that condition is good statistical hygiene," he says.

The results of scientific studies are reported in newspapers and magazines every day. It seems like the popular media is always pointing out something that might cause cancer. But some studies are more comprehensive and respected than others.

"Evidence accumulates," writes Walter C. Willett, M.D., in *Eat, Drink, and Be Healthy*, his book based on decades of nutritional research by the Harvard Medical School and Harvard's School of Public Health. "Like dropping stones onto an old-fashioned scale, the weight of evidence gradually tips the balance in favor of one idea over another. It is only when this happens that you should make changes in your life. The size of the stone clearly makes a difference.... Some types of studies are boulders, others are more like pebbles."

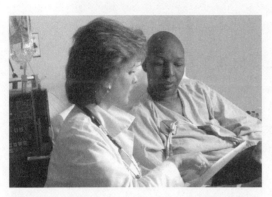

A doctor consults with a patient participating in a clinical trial. Photo courtesy of the National Cancer Institute Clinical Center and Mathews Media Group.

How to Tell If a Scientific Study Is the Final Word

So how do you know whom you can trust? The following are some issues to consider before you stop or start a behavior based on a study:

Where was the study originally reported? Well-known journals, such as the *New England Journal of Medicine, Science,* and the *Journal of the American Medical Association*, use strict peer-review criteria before they publish a study; that is, other scientists, researchers, and professionals review and critique the study before it is accepted for publication. This process lends more credibility to scientific reports.

Where did you read or hear about the study? Network news programs, national news magazines, and city newspapers are more likely to have science reporters who carefully translate scientific articles into reports for the general public. But, when working under tight deadlines, even experienced science reporters may be short on specifics.

Where was the research done? Most cancer research requires sophisticated scientific training, facilities, and equipment, so it's no surprise that most advances in cancer research come from well-known cancer centers, hospitals, and universities. Smaller hospitals and medical centers do generate valid research, but most research that has resulted in changes in clinical care are large, long-term studies carried out at major medical institutions.

Does the study support or contradict past research? One study that flies in the face of existing research may be more likely to make the headlines, but it's important to look at the big picture. The more evidence there is for something, the more likely it is to be valid.

Who were the research subjects? Some news items report studies from animal (or even test tube) research, which are important but not always immediately pertinent to humans. Sometimes specific ages and racial or ethnic groups are examined, such as African-American men over 75 with a high risk of prostate cancer or Ashkenazi Jewish women with a tendency to develop breast and ovarian cancers. Specific findings from such studies may not always apply to other groups of people.

What type of study was it? A *randomized controlled clinical trial*, where groups of individuals randomly assigned to different groups are compared, generally is considered the "gold standard" when it comes to evaluating effects on humans. (For more information on randomized controlled clinical trials, see page 81.)

How long did the study last? How large was it? Generally, studies affecting medical policy or guidelines are the result of years of research examining many people. It usually takes a number of such studies before the results are considered definitive.

Do you understand the terminology used in the study? Understanding the different implications of terms like *relative risk* and *absolute risk*, for example, is crucial in determining what study results mean for you. (For more about understanding risk terms, see *Risky Business* on pages 84–85.)

Are the study findings *statistically significant*? This term is a measurement to describe how often a particular result would occur simply by chance if the study or experiment were repeated many times. The most common minimum level accepted for statistical significance is 95 percent; meaning that if the study were repeated many times, the probability of this result occurring due to chance alone would be 5 percent or less.

Does the study promise a "magic bullet" for preventing or treating all cancers? Unfortunately, most beneficial changes can't be obtained easily with pills or potions. A healthy diet, exercise, and other good health habits are the best strategy for reducing a person's risk of cancer. Current cancer treatments are selected by doctors based on careful classification, or evaluation, of the type and extent of cancer in each patient. Claims of one treatment that cures all cases of all cancer types should be viewed skeptically.

Assessing Health-Related Web Sites

The growing specialty of science and health journalism is helping to create a bridge between researchers and the public. But the sheer volume of information available today through the Internet and other sources makes it increasingly challenging to sort the wheat from the chaff.

Web sites provide easy access to medical information, helping people to become more educated consumers. On the other hand, anybody can put up a Web site. Sometimes Web sites come across as more authoritative than they actually are.

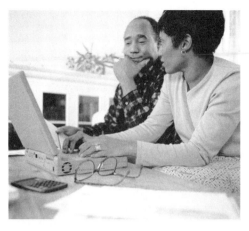

The Internet can deliver both solid medical data and false information. Sometimes it can be hard to tell the difference.

Many Web sites offer helpful, legitimate health-related information. But some Web sites present myths as facts, suggest unproven methods or miraculous cures, or offer opinions rather than scientific evidence. Sometimes it can be hard to tell the difference between respected sources and experimental ideas.

How can you figure out if a site reflects a respected source offering real health information? The NCI offers these ten ways to evaluate health information on Web sites:

1. Who runs the site? Any good health-related Web site should clearly state who is responsible for the site and its information.

2. Who pays for the site? The source of a site's funding should be clear. Are there advertisements on the site? If so, are they for respected products or services?

3. What is the purpose of the site? Check the "About This Site" link to see if it explains the goal of the site.

4. Where does the information come from? If the person(s) or organization in charge of the site didn't create the information, the original source should be labeled clearly.

5. What is the basis of the information? Medical facts and figures should have references. Opinions or advice should be set apart from information based on research results.

6. How is the information selected? Do people with excellent medical qualifications review the material before it is posted?

7. How current is the information? Medical information should be current and the site's most recent update or review date should be posted.

8. How does the site choose links to other sites? Some sites link only to other sites that have met certain criteria. Other Web sites link to any site that asks, or pays, for a link.

9. What information about you does the site collect and why? Any credible health sites asking for personal information about you should tell you exactly what they will and will not do with it. Be certain that you read and understand any privacy policy or similar language on the site.

10. How does the site manage interactions with visitors? There should always be a way for you to contact the site owners with problems, feedback, and questions.

Scientific Studies of All Shapes and Sizes

Scientific discoveries come about through experiments and studies. When you're considering the implications of a research study, it's a good idea to be able to tell *laboratory studies* from *human studies* and *observational studies* from *interventional studies*. If you understand the basics, you can evaluate study results more effectively.

Laboratory Studies

Laboratory studies, or test tube studies, are often the first step in cancer research. Researchers test substances on bacteria, animal, or human cells grown in laboratory dishes or test tubes. Animal studies may then help researchers learn more about a potential cancer-preventing substance or carcinogen's effects on a whole organism in a controlled environment.

Test-Tube Experimentation

In vitro (Latin for "in glass") studies use bacteria, animal, or human cells grown in laboratory dishes or test tubes. For example, the *Ames Test*, developed two decades ago by University of California at Berkeley biochemist Bruce N. Ames, shows whether a substance alters the DNA in bacteria. Researchers also sometimes add vitamins or other nutrients they suspect might protect DNA against cancer-causing mutations.

In vitro studies are often the first conducted after a potential cancer-causing (or cancer-preventive) agent is identified because they are easy to run, are relatively inexpensive, and take a short amount of time to complete. But they provide only a limited amount of information because they do not look at whole organisms.

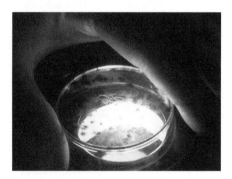

A technician adjusts a tissue culture dish under a microscope to measure the effects of chemicals on cultured cells. Photo courtesy of Linda Bartlett and the National Cancer Institute.

Mighty Mice

Once the stage is set through test-tube experimentation, highly specialized strains of mice perform for science. Modern lab mice are far more sophisticated than the plain white creatures that once dazzled scientists simply by finding their way through mazes.

Of Nude Mice and Men

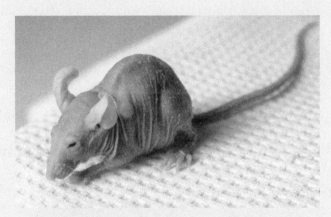

A genetically engineered nude mouse. Because of a genetic defect, nude mice have no thymus and cannot make certain cells essential for various immune responses. This characteristic makes them extremely helpful to scientists working in immunology research. Photo courtesy of Linda Bartlett and the National Cancer Institute.

The nude mouse gets its name because it has no hair. But more importantly, it is born without a thymus gland, which makes it unable to mount most types of immune responses.

Another mouse model has a deleted or "knocked out" *p53* gene — a tumor suppressor gene involved in more than half of human cancers — and is frequently used to screen for potential carcinogens.

In 2002, researchers developed a genetically altered mouse with two specific mutations that nearly always cause the mouse to develop *Rhabdomyosarcoma (RMS)*, and die soon after. This mouse represents the closest animal model for RMS, the most common soft-tissue childhood cancer, in humans to date. One of the mutations disrupts the proper development of muscle cells and tissue, but alone, rarely causes tumors to develop, while the other mutation interrupts a tumor suppressor function, and frequently results in human cancer. When the mutations are present together, their marked interaction offers the researchers an opportunity to learn more about the causes and development of this disease, as well as provide a prime target for testing potential therapies.

These humble, sometimes hairless animals are among the many mouse strains on the front lines of cancer research.

Today, scientists are using technology to modify the genes of mice and develop special strains, creating what are called *mouse models* for specific areas of cancer research. One mouse model, for instance, may be more susceptible to breast cancer while another mouse model is more sensitive to prostate cancer.

Animal studies are a major step beyond test tube studies and are a crucial component of cancer research. "If you can learn that something causes a mutation in an animal, it's more meaningful information than if it caused a mutation in bacteria," explains Harold Seifried, Ph.D., a program director in the Division of Cancer Prevention at the NCI.

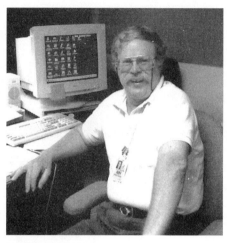

Harold Seifried, Ph.D.

Scientists can study the biological processes of every stage of tumor development by using laboratory animals. "[Animal studies] give you the big picture of the mechanisms of cancers and how they work in a whole animal, which is important," adds Seifried.

Unlike humans, animals can be studied in a well-controlled environment. Mice are especially valuable because they are similar to (although not the same as) humans in their genetic makeup and in their susceptibility to cancer. But tumors grow much more rapidly in mice than in humans—they develop within months, as opposed to years.

As valuable as the data gathered from mouse studies is, it is not all that's needed. A substance that causes cancer in mice, for example, may or may not cause cancer in humans, and the level of exposure needed to cause cancer may be far above any dose a person would be exposed to (as was the case with Alar).

"An animal study tells you if a compound has the potential to cause cancer, but not if it is a definite risk to humans," Seifried says. "There is a big difference. To determine whether something causes cancer, you need to get more than one piece of information."

But while animal studies cannot offer definitive proof of a cancer risk to humans, such studies can provide valuable information about where to focus research, continues Seifried. "If you give something to a mouse and it doesn't cause problems, you probably don't need to study it."

While hundreds of substances have been shown to cause cancer in laboratory animals, only a few dozen substances have been proven to cause cancer in humans. For many of them, such as asbestos and radium, the evidence came from high-dose occupational exposures. For obvious reasons, actual experiments that would subject humans to mega-doses of possible carcinogens cannot be carried out.

Human or Epidemiological Studies

Humans are much more difficult study subjects than laboratory animals for many reasons, including ethical ones. Most importantly, each person is different. Because of slight variations in individual genetic material, people come in an extraordinary array of colors, sizes, shapes—and susceptibility to different diseases.

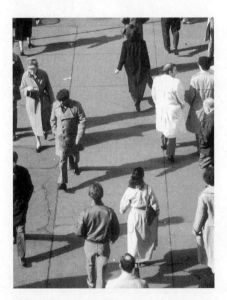

Epidemiologists study large groups of people, not individuals. Photo courtesy of Linda Bartlett and the National Cancer Institute.

But people don't only carry differences in their molecular makeups. Humans are also free-roaming, free-thinking organisms who vary their diets, exercise, and other day-to-day living patterns based on their age, sex, culture, and whims. They may live on farms or in skyscrapers. They may work on factory assembly lines or in air-conditioned banks. They may prefer a nondairy, no-carbohydrate diet or eat macaroni and cheese at every meal. Even people's constantly shifting moods and emotions play a role in their everyday biological functions.

Some daily habits—like how many packs of cigarettes a person smokes per day—are more easily measured. People tend to keep track of these types of habits. But when you ask someone to name everything they ate on an average day five years ago—or even last week—they are far less likely to give an accurate account.

The information gleaned from animal studies provides scientists with a sort of compass, as they wade into the much murkier, deeper waters surrounding the questions of what causes cancer in humans. The scientists who explore this territory are called epidemiologists.

"Epidemiology is endlessly fascinating and frustrating," asserts Patricia Hartge, Sc.D., the deputy director of the NCI's Epidemiology and Biostatistics Program. "What's so appealing about it is that by using relatively simple tools—like population statistics and other routine data—you can gain tremendous insights into biology."

As explained in chapter 2, epidemiologists focus on large groups of people, not individuals. Their studies of cancer risk estimate the likelihood of a certain part of a population developing cancer because of a particular exposure. But when epidemiologists estimate the risk related to an exposure, they usually need to describe the many uncertainties swirling around it.

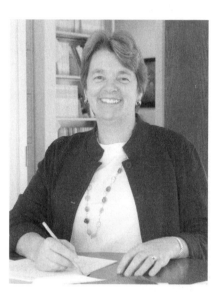

Patricia Hartge, Sc.D. Photo courtesy of Bill Branson and the National Cancer Institute.

"Every new finding in epidemiology raises many more questions that we are not able to answer," Hartge adds. "This is not the discipline for you if you want a [concrete] answer—the litmus paper doesn't turn either red or blue."

Inventiveness allows epidemiologists to think of new ways to ask questions about what is already known—and what is not known—in scientific literature. And humility is needed to seek input from specialists who might provide valuable clues to the meaning of a study's results.

"You can't know everything by yourself," says Hartge. "Epidemiology by nature is interdisciplinary. You often need to consult a geneticist or a physician in a particular field."

Epidemiological studies are categorized as observational or interventional based on the amount of involvement scientists have with the populations they study.

Observational Studies

Observational studies follow real people going about their normal lives, without any intervention from researchers. These kinds of studies often provide the first indication that something might cause (or prevent) cancer, and they are really the only way to determine if something causes cancer in humans. Observational studies are the most common type of epidemiological research and are broken down into three main categories:

1. *Ecological studies* compare the risk of a disease such as cancer in different populations. For example, these studies might tell researchers that lung cancer is more common in the United States and Western Europe than in most African countries. But they don't point to the specific factor or factors (like genetics, diet, smoking, or other environmental factors) that might cause it. Epidemiologists look for these differences, and then try to figure out if they actually play a role by using other kinds of studies.

2. *Case-control studies* often provide the first indication that something specific may be associated with an increased (or decreased) risk of a disease like cancer. These studies look at people (the "cases") with a certain type of cancer and then compare their histories to those of other people (the "controls") in similar situations who did not develop cancer. For example, case-control studies showing that smoking was more common

among people hospitalized for lung cancer than among patients in the same hospital for noncancerous problems were among the earliest evidence that smoking causes lung cancer.

3. *Cohort studies* follow a group of people (a "cohort") over a period of time. In most cohort studies, participants answer questions about exposures at the start of the study, before the researchers know who will eventually be diagnosed with a disease such as cancer. One of the strengths of cohort studies is that information about exposures is usually more accurate than in case-control studies. For example, some cohort studies ask participants to fill out a detailed record of what they eat over a certain period of time. This approach is more precise than asking people with a particular disease to recall what they regularly ate years earlier. The disadvantage of cohort studies is that they take much longer to complete than case-control studies do.

To conduct observational studies, investigators gather information about the behavior of a particular population through surveys and other methods. But they don't intervene or conduct experiments on people.

"Sometimes people, in effect, conduct experiments on themselves," says Hartge. "They decide if they will or will not smoke, or if they will or will not exercise. And we follow them and watch what happens and try to estimate the consequent risks."

Sometimes it appears that exposure to something in the environment has caused or prevented cancer. But a person's biological makeup can affect his or her development of cancer as well. Genetic and environmental variables are one of the greatest challenges to epidemiologists as they try to determine the likelihood of a single agent contributing to an increased—or decreased—risk of cancer.

The Sweet Truth

Sometimes, observational studies contradict previous laboratory findings. A 1972 laboratory study found that the artificial sweetener saccharin caused bladder cancer when given to rats in large doses. Most people don't consume more than moderate amounts of saccharin over extended periods, so epidemiologists didn't have a large group of humans to study.

Patricia Hartge, Sc.D., worked on an epidemiological study published in 1980 that showed that the level of saccharin used by most people did not cause an increase in bladder cancer. But for the handful of people involved in the study who consumed more than moderate amounts of saccharin, the data was less clear, suggesting that they may have a slightly increased risk for bladder cancer.

"At the end of the day, we found that if you are an average person who drinks moderate amounts of diet soda and occasionally uses saccharin, you don't have to worry," Hartge explains. "But if you are someone who drinks more than five diet sodas a day and you do that for 20 years, we don't know what that risk is. You can only study what people have done. Unlike an experiment, you can't make there be data when people have not created it."

For example, several observational studies have found that people who eat a high-fiber diet are less likely to develop colon cancer. But these studies don't tell us whether this statistical link reflects a direct result of eating fiber. In fact, most researchers now believe the reason these people develop colon cancer less often than those who don't eat a lot of fiber is that a high-fiber diet usually includes plenty of fruits and vegetables, which contain vitamins and countless other substances, one or more of which are probably responsible for reducing the risk of cancer.

Many epidemiological studies go on for years—sometimes even decades—before reaching a conclusive finding. Only occasionally is a finding immediately clear. An example of a sudden, dramatic correlation was the one drawn between vaginal cancer and *diethylstilbestrol (DES)*.

DES Exposure In Utero

DES was given to some pregnant women starting in the 1940s because it was believed to help prevent miscarriages. But in 1971, doctors made the observation that eight young women who had developed an extremely rare form of vaginal cancer had been exposed to DES while *in utero* (in the uterus). This was the first evidence that carcinogenic exposures could affect someone even before birth. Meanwhile, clinical trials had shown that DES did not reduce the chance of miscarriage.

The NCI is funding a long-term follow-up study on the women—and men—who were exposed to DES as fetuses. Even though the use of DES has been restricted, the follow-up study may yield answers to the question of how in utero exposures affect the risk of cancer later in life.

Interventional Studies

Because the conclusions that can be drawn from observational studies are often limited, researchers sometimes use interventional studies to try to confirm (or refute) their results.

With interventional studies, researchers intentionally change at least one factor they believe is related to the risk of a disease. These types of studies are the most likely to find a true link (or lack thereof) between something and cancer, but they can rarely be used for this purpose for ethical reasons.

Randomized controlled clinical trials are interventional trials where people are randomly assigned to one group or another, and some factor is intentionally kept different between the two. These are most often used to study new treatments but can also be used in prevention (in studying vitamin supplement use, for example.)

Randomized controlled clinical trials are the standard for study proof, but they are often difficult to run because of ethical concerns or cost. For example, it's virtually impossible to do a clinical trial to study the value of breast self-exams to detect breast cancer—it would be very difficult to find women who would be willing not to do them if they were randomly assigned to that group.

The HRT Bombshell

The Women's Health Initiative (WHI) was started in 1991 by the National Institutes of Health (NIH). One of the largest studies of women's health ever undertaken, the WHI is a randomized controlled clinical trial with more than 16,000 post-menopausal women ages 50 to 79 recruited to be in a variety of trials. The trials are designed to find ways to protect against major health risks facing these women, especially the number one killer, heart disease.

One part of the study, involving women taking a combination of estrogen and progestin hormones called *hormone-replacement therapy (HRT)*, was halted in July of 2002—three years earlier than planned. The findings for this study created a huge media sensation. It showed that HRT does not have protective benefits against heart disease, as observational data had indicated, but that it actually increases a woman's risk for heart disease. The interventional study also showed that HRT raises the risk for developing breast cancer.

Many of the six million women nationwide who have been taking HRT for years reacted angrily. How could their doctors have recommended a treatment that could harm their health in such serious ways?

"There are good reasons to explain why many physicians believed that HRT was beneficial to some postmenopausal women," states Eugenia Calle, Ph.D., director of analytic epidemiology at the ACS. "It's a great example of how difficult it can be to study something and what the limitations are."

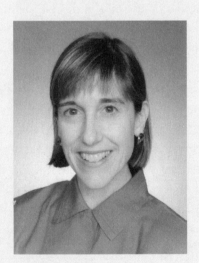

Eugenia Calle, Ph.D.

Decades ago when estrogen was first given to women to relieve menopausal symptoms, it became clear that it increased the risk for endometrial cancer. Progestin was added to the mix to help protect the endometrium. This so-called combination therapy, or HRT, appeared to have a complicated array of effects on the body. HRT seemed to have an impact on the heart and circulatory system, the bones, and cancers of the breast and colon.

"For years and years, observational studies of women who used hormones showed that, by and large, they were at decreased risk for heart disease and osteoporosis," Calle goes on to say. "The data on breast cancer was less clear. There was also a consensus that hormones lessened the risk for colon cancer."

The main problem in the observational studies was that they were not randomized studies—that is, they did not look at similar groups of women. In general, women who choose to take hormones tend to behave differently than those who do not. Overall they are leaner, are likely to see a doctor more regularly, and are less likely to smoke.

"A lot of work went into trying to eliminate this healthy-hormone-user effect, to come up with novel study designs and methods to deal with it," according to Calle. "These beliefs about the benefits of HRT were not made up out of whole cloth."

One way to eliminate the difference between hormone users and non-users was to conduct a randomized controlled clinical trial. About half of the 16,000 women involved in the HRT study were given HRT while the other half were given *placebos*, or dummy pills that have no effect.

Analysis of the results showed a slightly increased risk of invasive breast cancer, heart attacks strokes, and blood clots in the lungs for women taking HRT. Those same women taking HRT would benefit from a slightly decreased risk of colorectal cancer and hip fractures.

"Overall, the study findings suggested that the health 'costs' of taking HRT are greater than the benefits for the diseases examined. This was surprising. It was not something that either many women or physicians believed. But this is a situation where it was not anybody's fault for believing that," concludes Calle.

The study indicated that although the risks for breast cancer associated with HRT are small, they increase with every year of use. While HRT may still be appropriate for women who need short-term relief from menopausal symptoms, the WHI results changed the way we view long-term HRT use as a preventive agent for chronic diseases.

It's a good example of why rigorous scientific studies are needed to answer important medical questions.

Risky Business

Whether it's looking at the average daily temperature or considering your chances of winning the lottery, you encounter statistics in daily life. Statistics help researchers establish cancer risk as well. What we all ultimately want to know is, "What is my real risk of getting cancer?" Percentages and statistics can be misleading when it comes to cancer risk. Understanding study results and risk is all a matter of getting some context—having some knowledge in your back pocket.

Men rarely get breast cancer. But if you are a man, you might be alarmed to learn that a certain hypothetical substance increases your risk of breast cancer by 300 percent. You might be less worried about something hypothetical that increases your risk of prostate cancer by only 50 percent. But a man's risk of developing breast cancer in the first place is so low that tripling it isn't really changing it much at all. On the other hand, a man's risk of developing prostate cancer in his lifetime is fairly high to begin with (about one in six), so even a small change is significant.

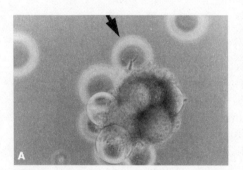 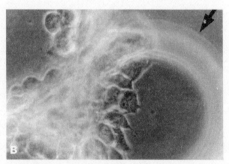

(A) Breast tumor cells aggregate where indicated by arrow. (B) The same image at higher magnification. Courtesy of Dr. Jeanne Becker, University of South Florida, and NASA's Marshall Space Flight Center.

So what do these risks really mean? Terms like lifetime risk, relative risk, and absolute risk are stumbling blocks for many laypeople.

Lifetime risk of cancer refers to the probability that an individual will develop cancer during his or her lifetime. In the United States, men have a one in two lifetime risk of developing cancer; for women the risk is one in three. The risk changes over the course of a person's life, generally lower when the person is younger and higher as the person grows older.

You'd probably be alarmed to read a headline stating that an everyday exposure doubles your risk of a certain type of cancer. Before refusing to leave the house, consider what type of risk the article is discussing. If you only have a one in one million lifetime risk of developing that type of cancer, and a factor doubles that to two in one million, that's still a very low risk.

Relative risk measures how strongly a particular risk factor influences the development of cancer (or a type of cancer). When determining relative risk, researchers consider one group's risk of developing cancer when exposed to a certain risk factor (like smoking) to the risk of another group without that risk factor (not smoking). Male smokers, for example, have about a 20-fold relative risk of developing lung cancer compared to nonsmokers. This means that smokers are about 20 times more likely to develop lung cancer than nonsmokers. Their risk is 2000 percent higher, but this still doesn't mean they will definitely develop the disease. Relative risk gives a sense of what will happen if one person is exposed to a risk factor and another is not.

Absolute risk, on the other hand, is the overall risk of developing cancer (or a type of cancer). By definition, your absolute risk for anything can only be between zero percent (no chance of developing the disease) and 100 percent (certainty you will develop the disease). In reality, however, the numbers are almost always somewhere in between. Absolute risk helps avoid overstating the dangers of a risk factor, especially if the risk of something happening is low. For instance, a factor may increase the relative risk of developing cancer by 100 percent. But if only one person in 100,000 currently develops that particular type of cancer, a 100 percent increase in risk means the factor is associated with two in 100,000 people developing cancer. The relative risk (100 percent) may sound large, but the absolute risk (.0002 percent) of one person developing cancer because of that risk factor may still be quite small.

Together, these three ways of considering cancer risk offer a balanced view of risk. Collecting and analyzing statistics can help researchers understand the possible relevance of the observations they're making. But individuals aren't populations, and cancer statistics only show cause or effect as related to large groups of people. Statistics don't predict what will happen to a particular person.

Making Informed Decisions

We are bombarded with messages these days that urge us to make constant assessments about our health and safety. It's not hard to find some kind of warning in the newspaper or on television telling you that the type of car you drive failed a crash test, or the prescription drug you take may have some serious side effects.

Most people's interest in knowing about research into the causes of cancer—or heart disease, or any other illness—boils down to this: What will increase my risk, and how worried should I be about it? For example, if you are exposed to a substance, will it increase the chances you'll develop cancer and if so, by how much? If you have a mutation in a gene associated with cancer, what are your odds of getting the disease? How will your everyday diet and exercise habits affect your cancer risk, and how much difference do they make?

"People really want to know, 'If I do something, what will be the benefit and what will be the harm?'" said Hartge. "It gets really challenging when you try to explain which associations [with cancer risk] are supported by strong evidence and which are supported by less strong evidence."

It is unlikely that exposure to any one factor will absolutely guarantee that you will or will not get cancer. But researchers try to provide people with guidelines so the public can assess the risks for themselves and make an informed decision.

When you're sorting through information about cancer risk, try to keep a steady course. Changing your life or expecting the worst because of a single study or news report will have you bouncing from one behavior to another every week. Each type of scientific study has its limitations, so it's important to consider a set of information over time rather than guiding your life based on a single study.

If you read or hear a report about cancer risk and you're interested in digging deeper than one reporter's account, consider taking a look at the study's abstract and summary for patients if it is provided. This is often an excellent overview of the study's important points and is written in an accessible way. Or turn to another trusted cancer information source, such as the ACS, the NCI, or other resources listed in the back of this book, for unbiased background information.

CHAPTER 5

The Dangers Around Us

I n the late 1980s, residents noticed that certain regions of Long Island, New York, had higher breast cancer rates than the national average. The island had been heavily farmed for many years but developed defense-related industries around the time of World War II. Some residents wondered whether pesticides and chemicals used in these industries might somehow have caused women in the area to get breast cancer.

People in the community brought attention to the issue and politicians paid attention. Although early pilot studies found no evidence of an environmental cause, pressure from activists led Congress to pass a law in 1993 that established the Long Island Breast Cancer Study Project. The project, funded by the National Cancer Institute (NCI) and the National Institute of Environmental Health Sciences, remains one of the largest studies ever undertaken to search for environmental factors that might trigger breast cancer.

The centerpieces of the project were case control studies on five environmental toxins, directed by Marilie Gammon, Ph.D., then at Columbia University and currently a University of North Carolina epidemiology professor.

In August 2002, Gammon released her study results. No connection was found between breast cancer and the now-banned pesticides DDT, chlordane, and dieldrin, or the banned group of industrial chemicals called *polychlorinated biphenyls (PCBs)*. (For more information on PCBs, see *The Truth about PCBs* on pages 98–99.) Only a very slight correlation was found between breast cancer and exposure to polycyclic aromatic hydrocarbons (PAHs), chemicals found in exhaust from cars, trucks, and aircraft and in cigarette smoke and grilled and smoked foods.

Some Long Island residents who pushed for years for the government to find answers to the elevated breast cancer rates felt let down when the study didn't answer their questions or confirm their fears.

"As a scientist, I think that I share that disappointment in the sense that when you spend many years doing a research project, you're always hoping that you're on the right path," Gammon told a news conference when she announced her team's study results. "There are many times we go up a particular pathway and it's not fruitful. There is still a lot [about] breast cancer that we cannot explain."

Elizabeth Ward, Ph.D., director of surveillance research for the American Cancer Society, notes, "The results of the Long Island study are consistent with the results of other studies that have examined the role of environmental contaminants in causing breast cancer. At the time the Long Island study was initiated, there was a great deal of concern that environmental contamination, especially with compounds such as DDT and PCBs, was responsible for the rising incidence of breast cancer in the United States as well as many other countries."

Presently, more than 25 studies on the subject have been completed, she notes. The studies have found no consistent relationship between chemicals such as DDT and PCBs and breast cancer risk.

Instead, reproductive factors may play a role in explaining increased breast cancer risk on Long Island and in similar communities. "Women in the Northeast tend to have children later and have fewer children than in the rural South, explains Francine Laden, Sc.D., an epidemiologist with Channing Laboratory at Harvard's Brigham and Women's Hospital in Boston who has been researching breast cancer and the environment since 1993. "These are known risk factors for breast cancer."

Environmental Causes of Cancer

When the average person talks about environmental factors, he or she is usually referring to air or water pollution. But to an epidemiologist, your *environment* is the combination of circumstances, physical conditions, and outside influences surrounding you. Any factor that is not inherited as part of your genetic makeup is environmental. Scientists generally agree that that most cancers arise from a combination of the genes we inherit and outside influences.

In this chapter, we'll discuss environmental hazards like cancer-causing chemicals and radiation that can affect large numbers of people in a community. In the following chapter, we'll look at potential cancer risks in the home and workplace, and we'll clarify which risks are genuine concerns and which ones you can safely ignore.

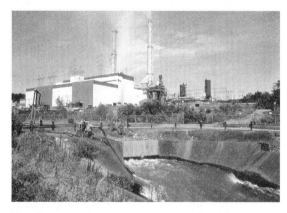

Laypeople tend to overestimate the cancer risk from environmental factors like air and water pollution. Photo courtesy of Linda Bartlett and the National Cancer Institute.

Putting Things in Perspective

Most experts believe that exposure to pollution and occupational and industrial hazards account for fewer than 10 percent of cancer cases. Smoking, for example, kills many more people than industrial chemicals or radiation.

But environmental risks sometimes seem scarier than known risk factors like poor diet, lack of exercise, and tobacco use. "If researchers tell us that alcohol causes oral cancer, which it does, then we can make an individual choice about whether to drink or how much to drink," says David Savitz, Ph.D., professor and chairman of the Department of Epidemiology at the University of North Carolina at Chapel Hill. "But when a cancer risk is something in the general environment, we don't have control over whether to accept or to not accept that risk."

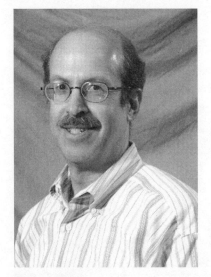

David Savitz, Ph.D.

For example, when members of the League of Women Voters and a group of college students were asked to prioritize their perceptions of their risk of death for 30 activities and technologies, both groups placed nuclear power first, ahead of smoking, drinking alcoholic beverages, and riding in motor vehicles. They perceived nuclear accidents and Chernobyl-type leaks as events with the highest risk of death. When professional risk experts ranked the actual risks based on recorded causes of death in the United States, smoking and motor vehicle accidents topped the list. Nuclear power was way down the list in twentieth place.

Savitz notes, "It's not very satisfying in some ways if people are concerned about pesticides and dump sites and pollution to steer cancer causes back to individual genes and behaviors. But more often you find that it's really pretty mundane, straightforward things that cause cancer, not exotic exposures like pollution."

Michael Thun, M.D., vice president of Epidemiology and Surveillance for the ACS, adds, "Pollution is an important problem in its own right, but the evidence that pollutants and pesticide residues increase the risk [of cancer] is presently quite weak and inconsistent. However, research into this area continues."

Cancer Clusters

A *disease cluster* is the occurrence of a greater than expected number of cases of a particular disease within a group of people, a geographic area, or a period of time. Notable disease clusters include the outbreak of Legionnaire's disease in the 1970s from contaminated water in air conditioning ducts, the initial cases of a rare type of pneumonia among homosexual men in the early 1980s that led to the identification of human immunodeficiency virus/acquired immune deficiency syndrome (HIV/AIDS), and periodic outbreaks of food poisoning caused by eating food contaminated with bacteria.

Cancer clusters may be suspected when people report that several coworkers, family members, friends, or neighbors have been diagnosed with the same or related cancers. In the 1960s, one of the best-known occupational cancer clusters emerged, involving an unusual number of cases of *mesothelioma* (a rare cancer of the lining of the chest and abdomen). Researchers traced the development of mesothelioma to exposure to a fibrous mineral called *asbestos*. Other notable cancer clusters in occupational settings include cases of lung cancer in underground uranium miners, bone cancer in radium watch dial painters, and an unusual form of lung cancer in workers exposed to vinyl chloride gas.

Cancer clusters in community (non-occupational) settings are typically more difficult to investigate and findings tend to be much less conclusive than investigations of concerns about cancer clusters in workplace settings. Currently, the Centers for Disease Control and Prevention (CDC) is investigating the causes of at least 16 cases of childhood leukemia since 1997 in Fallon, Nevada. Given a national average of about three childhood cases per 100,000 children, health officials report they would normally expect to see about one case every five years in Fallon, which has a population of 26,000. In May of 2002, two federal agencies ruled out the possibility of a jet fuel pipeline serving Fallon Naval Air Station as a public health hazard. In August 2002 the EPA launched a study to determine whether long-term exposure to arsenic in the drinking water has affected the health of the residents. Arsenic is a known human carcinogen—linked to skin, stomach, and bladder cancer although not associated with leukemia—and the city's water supply has arsenic levels of about 100 parts per billion, ten times the current standard.

"It's important to investigate cases like these," says David Schottenfeld, M.D., M.Sc., professor of epidemiology and internal medicine at the University of Michigan in Ann Arbor. But he adds that it is "very rare" for a cancer cluster to be scientifically linked to a specific environmental cause. "It's often not that simple and direct. The vast majority of cancer clusters are just random aberrations."

Most reported cancer clusters involve a variety of different kinds of cancer and cannot be shown to have a common cause. Before a cluster can be considered "true," epidemiologists must show that the number of cancer cases that have occurred is significantly greater than the number of cases that would be expected, given the age, gender, and racial distribution of the group of people at risk of developing the disease. A suspected cancer cluster is more likely to be a true cluster rather than a coincidence if it involves:

- many cases of a specific type of cancer, rather than several different types

- a rare type of cancer, rather than common types

- more cases of a certain type of cancer in an age group that is not usually affected by that type of cancer

Many reported clusters do not include enough cases to allow epidemiologists to arrive at any conclusions. "It's hard enough to prove the cause when you have [large numbers of cases], but with a small number of cases, it's even more difficult," notes Clark Heath, M.D., the former head of epidemiology for the ACS and one of the foremost experts on the subject. Sometimes, even when a suspected cluster has enough cases for study, epidemiologists can't prove a true statistical excess.

Other times, epidemiologists find an excess of cases but cannot find an explanation for the excess. There are currently no tests that determine the specific cause of cancer in an individual. The population may not be large enough to conduct a statistical study, and since it generally takes several decades for cancer to develop, there may not be records available to document what environmental contaminants were present in the past. Even when higher-than-expected levels of contaminants are found in the air, soil, or water of a community, it's difficult to tie exposure to one or more of the chemicals directly to increases in cancer.

Who Monitors What?

Food and Drug Administration (FDA) (*http://www.fda.gov*): The FDA regulates the safety of food (including labeling, additives, pesticide levels) and drugs, and medical and radiation-emitting devices (like cellular phones and microwaves), and it has limited authority over cosmetics as well.

Environmental Protection Agency (EPA) (*http://www.epa.gov*): The EPA is responsible for air, water, and food safety through the monitoring and control of environmental pollution.

Occupational Safety and Health Administration (OSHA) (*http://www.osha.gov*): A division of the U.S. Department of Labor, OSHA is responsible for creating and enforcing workplace safety and health regulations, including those relating to potential carcinogen exposures.

The Golden Rules of Toxicity

The earliest humans were hunters and gatherers and depended on nature to live. Today, many people in the United States spend most of their daily lives cut off from the elements, but human health is still closely tied to nature, according to Howard Frumkin, M.D., M.P.H., D.P.H., associate professor and chairman of environmental and occupational health at the Rollins School of Public Health at Emory University in Atlanta.

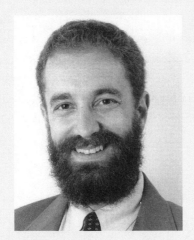

Howard Frumkin, M.D., M.P.H., D.P.H.

Frumkin cites studies showing that people exposed frequently to natural surroundings tend to be sick less and recover from ailments quicker. "People are resilient and they're also vulnerable," he remarks. "But the world is resilient and vulnerable too."

When the environment suffers, so do the people who live in it. The "six golden rules" of toxicity illustrate this correlation:

Rule 1: Toxins harm in predictable ways, and the more a person is exposed to the toxins, the harsher the reaction. However, carcinogens differ from other toxins in that being exposed to a higher dose of a carcinogen will increase your risk of developing a cancer, but it won't cause you to get a more aggressive cancer. That is why carcinogens are regulated differently than other hazardous substances.

Rule 2: Toxins can cause predictable reactions, but not everyone will react in the same way to them. For example, some people develop asthma when pollution is high, whereas others do not. Figuring out these inconsistencies is difficult but important, Frumkin notes, because it helps determine how society should regulate toxins.

Rule 3: Uncertainty is a fact of life. Most studies do not provide conclusive evidence of how the environment affects human health.

Rule 4: Despite the lack of conclusive evidence for some environmental toxins, society must do what it can to protect the environment, according to Frumkin. He cites the problem of global warming, which can cause more cholera, malaria, and flooding and less food production if left unchecked. Policy makers continue to debate this phenomenon, but Frumkin adds, "If we wait until we're 100 percent certain [of the problem], we may lose our chance to act."

Rule 5: Use an ounce of prevention. People should avoid toxins whenever possible to protect themselves, and society should protect the environment.

Rule 6: Environmental hazards do discriminate. Lower income areas may be more likely to become dumps for hazardous wastes.

Dump Sites and Pesticides

Toxic wastes in dump sites can threaten our health through air, water, and soil pollution. Laboratory experiments have shown many of the chemicals in toxic waste to be carcinogenic at high doses, but most communities appear to be exposed to low or negligible dose levels.

Pesticides and toxic chemicals can potentially cause health problems by polluting water. Chemical runoff from farm fields, yards, and golf courses treated with pesticides can contaminate streams and lakes, damaging natural food chains dependent on fish, shellfish, and other marine or freshwater life.

Groundwater contaminated by pesticides or other chemicals can also affect drinking water. Potential health risks are likely to be fewer now than in past years because pesticides that remain in the environment (such as DDT) have been largely replaced by products that are quickly degraded. Thanks to water treatment processes, dangerous levels of suspected carcinogens in the water system are rare.

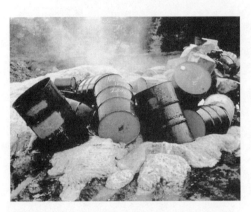

Toxic materials in dump sites are environmental hazards. Photo courtesy of *http://www.whitehouse.gov*.

The level of exposure is key to assessing risks, explains Savitz. For pesticides, the at-risk population "is really the people who mix and apply the pesticides, not the people buying an apple at the store," he concludes.

The Truth about PCBs

Polychlorinated biphenyls (PCBs) are a group of more than 200 related chemicals that were used by U.S. industries from the 1930s until they were banned in the late 1970s. PCBs were used industrially and commercially in hundreds of ways, including in electrical, heat transfer, and hydraulic equipment; as plasticizers in paints, plastics, and rubber products; and in dyes and carbonless copy paper. Congress banned PCBs in 1976 because of concern about the toxicity of PCBs and their impact on the environment.

We now know that PCBs cause cancer in animals. The EPA and the International Agency for Research on Cancer (IARC), part of the World Health Organization (WHO), consider PCBs a probable cause of cancer in humans.

PCBs are still in the environment. PCBs continue to be released from leaking old equipment, from leaching landfills, and from previously contaminated deposits. Minute amounts of PCBs are in most

How Are Carcinogens Classified?

Several monitoring and regulatory groups consider similar criteria to find out if an agent is carcinogenic. The most widely used system employed to answer the question of "Will this substance cause cancer?" comes from the International Agency for Research on Cancer (IARC). It divides agents into general categories: substances that definitely cause cancer in humans; substances that probably cause cancer; substances that possibly cause cancer; substances for which the cancer risk is unknown; and substances that are probably not cancer causing. The IARC's monographs evaluating carcinogenic risks of substances to humans can be found online at *http://monographs.iarc.fr/*.

It may not be surprising that most of the 750 or so agents listed by the IARC are of possible/probable or unknown risk. There is just not enough strong evidence to determine if many substances definitely do or definitely do not cause cancer. About 50 are classified as carcinogens.

In the United States, the National Toxicology Program (NTP), formed from parts of several government agencies (including the NIH, CDC, and the FDA), creates a *Report on Carcinogens* every few years, which classifies "known human carcinogens" or "reasonably anticipated human carcinogens." Examples of familiar substances known to cause cancer in humans include arsenic, asbestos, radon, tobacco smoke, and smokeless tobacco. Over 200 agents appear on this list. You can find the complete list of carcinogens and more information about the NTP on its Web site: *http://ntp-server.niehs.nih.gov/NewHomeRoc/AboutRoC.html*.

foods, water supplies, and the air. Most people are exposed to PCBs by consuming food or water from contaminated areas. But there's no reason to panic: in general, the levels of PCBs found in drinking water and the air are low and insignificant, and the concentrations of PCBs in food are many thousand times below the concentrations that have been shown to cause cancer in animal experiments.

Radiation

For some people, the word "radiation" conjures up powerful images of nuclear reactors and technicians suited in head-to-toe protective gear to work with radioactive materials. But *radiation* is the emission (sending out) of energy from any source, including the light that comes from the sun and the heat coming from our bodies.

Only high frequency radiation (*ionizing radiation* and *ultraviolet radiation*) has been proven to cause cancer. Most forms of radiation are *nonionizing* (that is, don't have the energy to cause DNA damage) and have not been clearly linked to cancer.

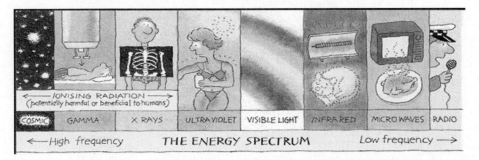

Reprinted from *Radiation and Life* Web graphic by permission of Uranium Information Centre, Ltd., Melbourne, Australia. Available at: *http://www.uic.com.au/ral.htm*. Accessed December 23, 2002.

Types of ionizing radiation include x-rays, gamma rays, cosmic rays, and particles given off by radioactive materials, like alpha particles, beta rays, and protons. People may be exposed to the following main sources of ionizing radiation:

- *Natural background radiation* comes from cosmic rays in outer space and from radioactive elements normally present in the soil, such as radon. Natural background radiation is the major contributor to worldwide radiation exposure.

- *Nonmedical synthetic radiation* occurs as a result of above-ground nuclear weapons testing that took place before 1962, as well as occupational and commercial sources.

- *Medical radiation* comes in the form of diagnostic x-rays and other tests, as well as from radiation therapy. *Radiation therapy* is currently used to treat some types of cancer and involves dosages many times higher than those used in diagnostic x-rays. (For more information, see the *Medical Radiation* section on pages 117–119 of this chapter.)

- Ultraviolet radiation (sometimes called UV radiation) comes from exposure to sunlight (and tanning lamps) and causes almost all cases of skin cancer.

Nonionizing Radiation

Certain forms of radiation have not been clearly linked to cancer but still get a lot of attention. Because of their low frequencies, these nonionizing forms of radiation don't have the energy to cause DNA damage. Forms of nonionizing radiation include microwaves, radio waves, and radar, as well as *electromagnetic radiation*—a type of nonionizing radiation produced by moving electric charges, found in power lines and electronic devices such as cellular phones and televisions.

Although some studies have suggested associations between nonionizing radiation and cancer, most of the now-extensive research in this area does not. Furthermore, it has been difficult to figure out a way that this type of radiation could cause cancer.

"Electromagnetic radiation is a type of radiation, and radiation is a scary subject to a lot of people. There's a lot of concern about things that you can't see," remarks Joseph Fraumeni, Jr., M.D., M.Sc., director of the Division of Cancer Epidemiology and Genetics at the National Cancer Institute in Bethesda, Maryland. He notes that the growing body of epidemiological evidence suggests that the fears regarding electromagnetic radiation are blown out of proportion.

"There is always the possibility that the studies haven't been big enough, they haven't gone on long enough, or that the risks are so low that they are very, very difficult to detect," he speculates. Research—and controversy—in this area continues.

Electromagnetic Fields

In 1999, the National Institute of Environmental Health Sciences (NIEHS) released the results of an extensive six-year study. It stated that the evidence for a risk of cancer and other human disease from the *electric and magnetic fields (EMF)* around power lines is "weak" at best but could not totally be discounted, and that efforts to reduce exposures when possible should continue.

Recent extensive studies of electric utility workers showed a minimal increase in their risk of brain tumors and leukemia, but these increases were so small that it is almost impossible to determine if electromagnetic fields were truly the cause. Results from some studies on magnetic fields and childhood leukemia have suggested a link but have been inconsistent. Smaller studies have linked cancer and activities like using electric blankets and watching television, but the most recent and largest study did not find a connection between electromagnetic fields and cancer.

The conflicting data and controversy about electromagnetic fields will undoubtedly continue until the question of whether electromagnetic fields can cause cancer is answered.

"Controversy often occurs when we're trying to discriminate between no increase in risk and a tiny increase in risk," according to Savitz. "People want absolute terms."

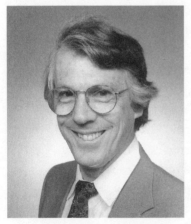

Michael Thun, M.D.

Cellular Phones

Recent media attention has focused on a possible link between cellular phone use and brain cancer. Cellular phones operate with radio frequencies (RF) and do not emit ionizing radiation, the type that damages DNA. But researchers admit that since cell phones are relatively new, no long-term follow-up studies on their possible biological effects exist. "Assessing the health risks of a new technology is always a dilemma," says ACS's Thun. "Because cellular telephone technology is new, data from large studies are not yet available on long-term use."

While most evidence from animal and human studies to date points to no association between brain tumors and cell phones, an occasional study does show what appears to be a potential risk.

A Finnish government agency announced in June 2002 that an animal study suggested that mobile phone emissions might affect the cells that control the biochemical barrier between the blood and the brain. That could make the barrier more permeable and could be dangerous.

But one of the Finnish researchers cautioned the public not to jump to conclusions. The study was designed to show whether cell phones caused *biological* effects, but it did not provide information about possible *health* effects. "This is a new technology and we should evaluate the health aspects properly, but we shouldn't blow the concern out of proportion," says John Boice, Sc.D., scientific director of the International Epidemiology Institute in Rockville, Maryland.

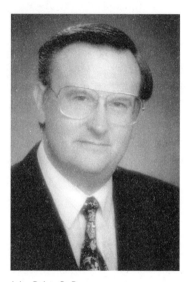

John Boice, Sc.D.

Thun agrees, adding that the lack of ionizing radiation and the low-energy level emitted from cell phones and absorbed by human tissues make it unlikely that these devices cause cancer.

Moreover, several well-designed epidemiological studies find no consistent association between cell phone use and brain cancer. For example, one study of adult cell phone users with and without brain tumors found that regardless of years of use or number of minutes of use per day reported, there was no increased risk of brain tumors for cell phone users compared to nonusers. Brain tumors also did not occur more frequently on the side of the head where cell phone users reported holding their phone.

The FDA Center for Devices and Radiological Health has stated, "If there is a risk from these products—and at this point we do not know that there is—it is probably very small." If you are concerned about avoiding even *potential* risks, the FDA recommends you switch to a car phone with an antenna outside the vehicle or a headset plugged into a cellular phone carried at the waist.

Invisible Intruder: Radon

Most lung cancer cases are directly related to smoking. But the number two culprit for lung cancer is *radon*, a colorless, odorless gas that occurs naturally in soil, rocks, underground water, and air. It's produced by the *radioactive decay* (natural breakdown) of uranium in soil and rocks. Then radon breaks down further into decay products that attach to particles in the air. Outdoor radon levels are minute. But when radon enters a building—or your home—its decay products can accumulate.

"The vast majority of homes in the United States are at a reasonable level [of radon] and are nothing to be concerned about," says Boice. "But if there is a high reading, it could be a serious health hazard. It's always good to conduct a test. There is no sense in being in a home and breathing high levels of radon unnecessarily."

Major health organizations, including the ACS, agree that radon causes thousands of preventable lung cancer deaths every year, even in nonsmokers. Smokers exposed to high levels of radon in their homes have even higher risks for lung cancer than other smokers. When inhaled, radon decay products become trapped in the lungs, where the ionizing radiation energy is believed to begin the gradual cancer-causing process.

Radon levels are highest in the Northeast and Midwest, but high radon levels have been found in every state and vary from area to area. Your home may have a high radon level, yet your neighbor's may be within acceptable limits. Radon is measured in picocuries per liter (pCi/L), and the EPA urges anyone whose level at home is above 4 pCi/L (an estimated 8 million American homes) to take action. By comparison, the average outdoor air radon level is about

0.4 pCi/L, although it can be higher in certain areas.

An airtight home with all cracks carefully sealed keeps warm air in during the winter. It also allows radon to accumulate year-round. But radon can be present in any home. Until you test, you simply don't know if your radon level is high.

Both short- and long-term tests are available and are relatively inexpensive (less than 50 dollars). The National Safety Council (NSC) operates a Radon Hotline (800-557-2366) to answer questions and provide materials about radon, its health effects, and

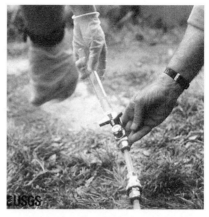

Water for radon measurements is collected at a well head through a diaphragm designed to keep the water sample from coming into contact with air or being exposed to light. Photo courtesy of the United States Geological Survey, *http://az.water.usgs.gov/cazb/pix/radon.jpeg.*

radon testing. Listings of contractors qualified to conduct radon testing and make home modifications to lower radon levels are available on the EPA Web site at *http://www.epa.gov/iaq/contact.html.* Each state also has a radon information office with a list of approved testing companies.

The following are suggestions for testing radon in your home:

- Before you buy a home, insist that it be tested. Be suspicious of cracked foundations or homes with crawl spaces under family rooms or bedrooms.

- Before you sell your home, test it to assure potential buyers that the radon level is low.

- If your radon test registers above 4 pCi/L, you can take action to lower the radon level. You may be able to install pipes and fans below concrete floors and foundations or put a fan in your crawl space to vent the area.

- Include radon-resistant techniques in your building plans for renovating, finishing your basement, or for new construction.

Exposing the Sun

Ultraviolet radiation is a stream of high-energy rays from the sun that can damage DNA—both in the skin and eyes. Although it is a component of sunlight, UV radiation is not visible to the naked eye. The amount of UV rays a person is exposed to depends on the strength of the sunlight, the amount of time exposed, and whether his or her skin and eyes are protected.

Some forms of high-energy radiation, including UV rays, can damage DNA at a cellular level. This damage can make DNA less able to control how and when a cell grows and divides. Changes in DNA, called mutations, seem to be a necessary part of the development of cancer; although in most cases it probably takes more than just one mutation to cause cancer. Some people are born with DNA mutations inherited from their parents, which make them more likely to develop cancer. This explains why one person may be more likely to develop skin cancer than another, even if both are exposed to the same amount of UV rays.

Ultraviolet radiation is actually divided into three wavelength categories:

- *UVA rays* are not absorbed by the ozone layer. They travel from the sun straight to the Earth—and our bodies. They are involved in the aging of cells and produce some damage to DNA.

- *UVB rays* are partially absorbed by the ozone layer. They are mainly responsible for direct damage to DNA and are thought to cause most skin cancers.

- *UVC rays* do not reach Earth because they are completely absorbed by oxygen and ozone in the atmospheres, so they pose no risk to humans.

There are no safe UV rays.

Skin cancer is the most common—and one of the most preventable—of all cancers. More than 90 percent of skin cancers develop on sun-exposed skin: face, neck, forearms, and hands.

More than one million cases of skin cancer are reported in the United States each year. The most common type of skin cancer, *nonmelanoma*, can be classified as either *basal cell* or *squamous cell* cancer. Basal cell cancer begins in the lowest layer of the epidermis, called the basal cell layer. About 75 percent of all skin cancers are basal cell cancers. Squamous cell cancers come from the higher levels of the epidermis and account for about 20 percent of all skin cancers. In most cases, nonmelanoma skin cancer is highly curable, but more than 2,000 people are expected to die from it this year.

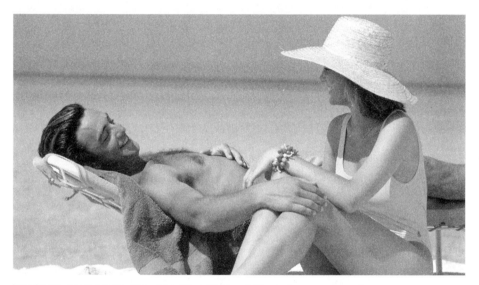

Harmful sun rays can cause skin cancer—the most preventable, most common type of cancer.

Melanoma (cancer that starts in the *melanocytes*, or pigment-producing cells) is a much more serious form of skin cancer. Melanoma accounts for only about 4 percent of skin cancers overall but causes about 79 percent of skin cancer deaths. An estimated 7,400 people will die this year from melanoma.

Melanoma incidence has skyrocketed in the United States. Since 1973, the number of new cases for melanoma has more than doubled, and the number of deaths caused by melanoma has increased by nearly 44 percent. The death rates from melanoma are increasing most rapidly among white men 50 years and older.

Are You Exposed?

The amount of UV radiation that reaches Earth depends on the following factors:

- **Closeness to the equator.** At the equator the intensity of the sun is naturally stronger because of its location directly overhead. Not only do the sun's rays have less distance to travel, but the ozone layer is also thinner in the tropics.

- **Altitude.** Ultraviolet rays are stronger at higher altitudes because there is less atmosphere to absorb the damaging radiation. The risk of overexposure to UV rays is greater the higher you go, which explains why skiers and other mountain-sports enthusiasts must do more to protect their skin.

- **Time of day.** The sun's rays travel at an angle early in the morning and late in the afternoon, thereby reducing the intensity of damaging UV light. The sun is at its highest point in the sky around noon. At this time UV light has less atmosphere to travel through and less distance to travel.

- **Time of year.** The sun's angle to Earth changes with the seasons, resulting in changes in UV intensity. UV rays are strongest in late spring and early summer.

- **Weather.** UV rays can reach you even on cloudy days. Although UV levels are reduced on cloudy days, it is possible to burn your skin even if the cloud cover is thick. Overcast days are especially dangerous because many people feel they are safe from the sun's harmful effects, so they don't bother to protect themselves.

- **Mirroring.** The sun reflects off many surfaces, including water, sand, concrete, grass, and snow. UV light can also reach below the water's surface. Even in shaded areas it's important to be aware of reflection.

- **Ozone layer.** The ozone layer is in a region of the upper atmosphere called the stratosphere. It absorbs most UVB and all UVC radiation coming from the sun, but it does not absorb UVA radiation. The ozone layer has become thinner due to the release of ozone-depleting substances widely used in industry. The thinner ozone has allowed more of the sun's ultraviolet radiation to reach Earth.

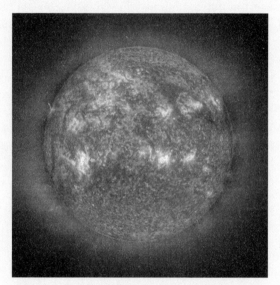

An image of the sun taken by the Solar and Heliospheric Observatory's Extreme-Ultraviolet Imaging Telescope. Image courtesy of the EIT Consortium, the National Aeronautics and Space Administration (NASA), and the National Space Science Data Center (NSSDC).

To increase awareness of the damaging potential of UV radiation, the EPA and the National Weather Service (NWS) developed the *UV Index*. It predicts the probable intensity of UV radiation reaching Earth's surface during the sun's peak (usually around noon).

The UV Index is expressed as a number ranging from 0 to 10+ that indicates the amount of UV radiation reaching Earth's surface around noon each day. The higher the UV Index number, the greater the risk for exposure to UV radiation and the less time it takes before skin damage occurs.

The Sunscreen Scene

Summer sunburn has become the norm for people ages 11 to 18, according to a 1999 study done by Alan Geller, R.N., M.P.H., and associates from Boston University and Harvard Medical School, both in Boston, and the Memorial-Sloan Kettering Cancer Center in New York.

People are very aware of the fact that exposure to UV rays can lead to skin cancer, but following the recommendations for protecting skin are a challenge for many people. For example, many people apply sunscreen too thinly. Others may not apply it at all to avoid feeling greasy, getting sunscreen in their eyes, or clogging their pores. Still others apply sunscreen initially, but forget to reapply it after swimming or perspiring.

It is especially important for adults to take special care with children, because children tend to spend more time outdoors and can burn more easily. Hats that protect the ears and neck, long-sleeved shirts and pants, sunglasses that block 100 percent UVA and UVB rays, and sunscreens that block both UVA and UVB rays and have a *sun protection factor (SPF)* of 15 or more help protect skin and eyes from the sun. The majority of sun exposure occurs before the age of 18 for most people; studies increasingly suggest a link between early exposure and the development of skin cancer as an adult.

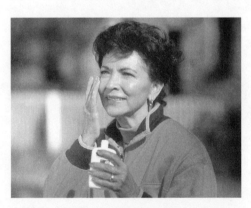

Applying sunscreen before going outdoors and then reapplying it at regular intervals can help prevent skin cancer. Photo courtesy of Bill Branson and the National Cancer Institute.

Who's at Risk?

Everyone's skin and eyes are susceptible to sun damage. Although people with light skin are more vulnerable, darker-skinned people, including African Americans and Hispanic Americans, also can be affected. Skin type—not race or ethnicity—is the key question when considering the sun's effect on an individual.

Skin Type and Sunburn Risk

Skin Type	Tanning and Sunburning History
I	Always burns, never tans, sensitive to sun exposure
II	Burns easily, tans minimally
III	Burns moderately, tans gradually to light brown
IV	Burns minimally, always tans well to moderately brown
V	Rarely burns, tans profusely to dark
VI	Never burns, deeply pigmented, least sensitive

Reprinted from Choose Your Cover, Centers for Disease Control and Prevention, National Center for Chronic Disease Prevention and Health Promotion, Division of Cancer Prevention and Control, 2000.

People with skin types I and II are at the highest risk for skin cancer as a result of excessive sun exposure, but people of all skin types can develop skin cancer.

People with darker skin have more melanin, a naturally protective pigment, and they tan more easily than others. Melanin in the skin helps block out damaging rays to a certain extent, which is why darker-skinned people burn less easily. But contrary to popular belief, people with darker skin are not completely protected from sun damage and skin cancer. Individuals with the following conditions are at higher risk:

- lots of moles, irregular moles, or large moles

- a previous diagnosis of skin cancer

- an indoor lifestyle during the week and intense sun exposure on weekends

- a primarily outdoor lifestyle

- a home or vacation destination in a tropical or subtropical climate or at high altitudes

- a tendency to burn before tanning

- fair skin, freckles, or blond, red, or light-brown hair

- a family history of skin cancer, especially melanoma

- an organ transplant

- certain diseases, such as lupus, that increase sensitivity to the sun

- certain long-term severe skin problems, such as serious burns or psoriasis (an inflammatory skin disease) that have been treated with UV light

- radiation treatment or exposure to arsenic

- medications that increase sensitivity to the sun, such as: antibiotics, ibuprofen, major tranquilizers and anti-nausea drugs, antidepressants, and chemotherapy agents.

Tanning Salons

Many people are under the impression that tanning using a sunlamp or tanning bed is safer than natural sunlight. But a single 15- to 30-minute session in a tanning salon exposes the body to the same amount of harmful UV sunlight as a full day at the beach, according to experts.

A recent study by Vilma Cokkinides, Ph.D., and colleagues from the ACS and Brown University in Providence, Rhode Island, looked at the use of sunlamps by young people aged 11 to 18 in the United States. They also looked at the tanning behavior of the young people's parents.

They found that if a parent used a sunlamp in the previous year, 30 percent of their children did the same. More disturbing, they say, was the finding that four of ten young women aged 17 and 18 used a tanning sunlamp during the previous year.

Other factors associated with the use of tanning lamps, aside from age and parental influence, included a desire to be tan and not using a sunscreen of 15 or higher when at the beach or pool.

Medical Treatments

Some medical treatments are powerful enough to alter DNA and cause cancer themselves. Often the benefits of using these treatments far outweigh the potential risks, as in the case of chemotherapy. The risks and benefits of other treatments, such as hormone therapy, may be more complicated.

Chemotherapy

You might not know you're being exposed to a chemical carcinogen like arsenic. Those who undergo *chemotherapy*, on the other hand, are exposed to the powerful chemicals to treat a disease that has already been diagnosed. Over one hundred chemotherapy drugs are currently used to destroy cancer cells—either alone or in combination with other treatment. And many more are expected to become available. Chemotherapy, the primary method for treating many cancers, is often used with surgery or radiation to treat cancer that has spread (metastasized), cancer that has come back, or if there is a strong chance that it could come back.

Chemotherapy, unlike surgery or radiation, is a systemic therapy. This means that the medicines travel throughout the body, or system, rather than being confined or localized to one area of the body. Because chemotherapy can kill cancer cells that may have metastasized to other parts of the body, it is often the most effective form of treatment for cancer that has spread.

Another cancer sometimes develops because of chemotherapy treatment. These secondary cancers can include *Hodgkin's disease* and non-Hodgkin's lymphoma, *leukemias*, and some solid tumors.

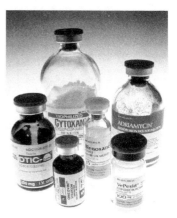

Chemotherapy is the primary method for treating many cancers. Photo courtesy of the National Cancer Institute.

The cancer risk is greater with some chemotherapy drugs than with others. For this reason, and because of these drugs' other adverse effects, oncologists do not recommend chemotherapy unless they have good reason to believe it will help the patient, and the benefit will far outweigh the risk of a second cancer later on.

Hormones

Hormones have been used to treat and prevent certain diseases for decades. Many cancers, including cancers of the breast, cervix, uterus, and ovaries, grow in response to hormones. And in the cases of diethylstilbestrol (DES), hormone replacement therapy (HRT), oral contraceptives, and *Tamoxifen* (a drug used to treat breast cancer), the use of hormones may increase a woman's risk of developing certain types of cancer. In contrast, these medications can also be used to prevent, or even treat, some cancers.

Hormone replacement therapy (HRT) went from medical acceptance to medical uncertainty in a heartbeat in 2002 when researchers reported that it increases the risk of breast cancer, heart attacks, strokes, and blood clots. They immediately cautioned healthy women against continuing or starting long-term use of HRT to prevent heart disease.

But despite the alarm, women should still consider the researchers' complete recommendations and talk with their own doctors before deciding whether HRT is friend or foe. It may still be a useful short-term option to treat the symptoms of menopause. The increased risks for an individual woman are still quite small.

"Decisions to take hormone replacement therapy, particularly *estrogen* plus *progestin*, which is widely prescribed, will be more difficult now," said Harmon Eyre, M.D., chief medical officer for the ACS.

The findings about HRT came from the Women's Health Initiative (WHI), a long-term study of more than 16,000 healthy, postmenopausal women funded by the NIH. The results were published in the July 17, 2002 *Journal of the American Medical Association*. (For more information about the design of the study, see pages 82–83.)

The women began taking either a combination estrogen/progestin pill or a placebo each day, starting in the mid-1990s.

After five years, directors stopped the study early because the risks of HRT outweighed and outnumbered the benefits. This long-term use of oral estrogen/progestin therapy led to the following health problems—and some benefits:

- a 26 percent increase in breast cancer, but no increase in breast cancer deaths

- a 41 percent increase in strokes

- a 29 percent increase in heart attacks

- doubled rates of blood clots in legs and lungs

- 37 percent decrease in colorectal cancer

- 34 percent fewer hip fractures and 24 percent fewer total fractures

Individual Risks Are Small

Women should not be alarmed by the statistics above. A 26 percent increase in a small risk for breast cancer is still a small risk. "Each woman in the study who took the estrogen plus progestin therapy had an increased risk of breast cancer of less than a tenth of one percent per year," according to a statement from the WHI. Among 10,000 women taking HRT, in a single year there would be 38 women diagnosed with breast cancer, compared with 30 diagnoses of breast cancer among women not taking HRT.

The study results do not apply to women receiving only *estrogen replacement therapy (ERT)*, still commonly given to women who have had a hysterectomy. The effects of ERT on women who no longer have a uterus are being studied in a separate WHI clinical trial, with results expected in 2005.

In the United States, 38 percent of menopausal women take some form of HRT—for several different reasons. Women find it especially effective in treating hot flashes, sleeplessness, moodiness, and other disruptive symptoms of menopause. It also helps prevent osteoporosis. And until now, HRT has been touted as a way to help prevent heart disease well after menopause.

What Women Should Do Now

WHI researchers made the following specific recommendations on what to do now:

- The therapy should not be continued or started to prevent heart disease. Women should consult their doctor about other methods of prevention, such as lifestyle changes and cholesterol- and blood pressure—lowering drugs.

- For osteoporosis prevention, women should consult their doctor and weigh the benefits against their personal risks for heart attack, stroke, blood clots, and breast cancer. Alternate treatments also are available to prevent osteoporosis and fractures.

- Women should keep up with their regular schedule of mammograms and breast self-examinations.

- Although short-term use was not studied, women taking the therapy for relief of menopausal symptoms may reap more benefits than risks. Women should talk with their doctor about their personal risks and benefits.

Drugs used for many years must meet high standards for safety, especially when they're taken by healthy people to keep them that way. Two independent experts, Suzanne Fletcher, M.D., M.Sc., and Graham Colditz, M.D., M.P.H., both of Harvard Medical School emphasize this in an editorial about the WHI study: "Given these results, we recommend that clinicians stop prescribing this combination for long term use. *'Primum non nocere'* [First, do no harm] applies especially to preventive health care."

Medical Radiation

As with chemotherapy, certain forms of medical radiation can lead to an increased risk of cancer. The benefits of using these types of medical radiation, however, generally far outweigh the risks associated with them.

Radiation Therapy

Radiation therapy uses high-energy ionizing radiation to destroy cancer cells and treat or control cancer. Radiation therapy's cancer-causing potential was recognized many years ago. In fact, much of our knowledge about ionizing radiation has come from studying the survivors of the atomic bombs and their radiation in Japan, from workers' occupational exposure to radiation, and from patients treated with radiation therapy for malignant and nonmalignant disease.

Despite being relatively rare, the development of a second cancer is more common among those who receive radiation therapy than those who do not.

"It's a fine balance," says Boice, an expert on ionizing radiation. "You have to weigh the risk against the medical benefit. If you have a cancer and you're going to be treated with radiation, you should be concerned about the risk of developing a second cancer, but not to the extent that you turn down possible treatment. On the other hand, you should certainly discuss the treatment options fully with your doctor."

Most cases of leukemia related to radiation exposure develop within a few years of exposure, peaking at five to nine years then slowly declining. Most other forms

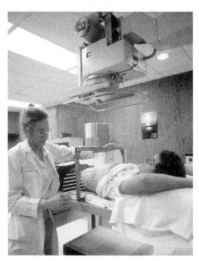

A technician prepares a person with cancer for radiation therapy. Photo courtesy of Linda Bartlett and the National Cancer Institute.

of cancer do not occur until ten years after radiation exposure, and some cancers are diagnosed even fifteen or more years later. Radiation-related leukemia risk depends on a number of factors, such as the amount of radiation received, the percentage of bone marrow exposed to radiation, and whether the patient was also treated with chemotherapy.

Studies of radiation-related breast cancer have found the greatest risk in women who were irradiated as children and adolescents for other conditions. (The most common reason for adolescents to have chest radiation is Hodgkin's disease, a type of lymphoma.) Oncologists (doctors specializing in cancer treatment) know about the increased risk of breast cancer in these women and generally recommend that they have vigilant lifetime screening for breast cancer. However, according to Boice, most studies of individuals with Hodgkin's disease have found no increased breast cancer risk among women who receive radiation at 30 years and older.

X-rays and Mammography

Many people are concerned about their exposure to x-rays. X-rays (including *mammograms*, x-rays of the breast) use doses of radiation that are many times lower than those used in radiation therapy. As with radiation therapy, studies in the past have shown that there appears to be some risk in receiving many x-ray examinations, particularly for children who have multiple x-rays. The level of radiation in modern x-rays is much lower than that used even 25 years ago and poses much less of a risk. While it's a good idea to minimize repeat exposures whenever possible, especially in children, it's important not to avoid necessary x-rays.

The dose of radiation received by women over 40 during modern mammograms does not significantly increase their risk for breast cancer. To put this dose into perspective, a woman who receives radiation as a treatment for Hodgkin's disease might receive several thousand *rads* (the unit of radiation dose). A single mammogram is much less than 1 rad. Further, exposures later in life, even at high doses, are associated with a very low future risk.

CT Scans

Computed tomography (CT) scans use larger doses of radiation than those found in conventional x-rays. Again, concern has been raised over the possibility of an increased cancer risk in children who receive multiple CT scans. Ways to lower radiation doses without compromising medical value are encouraged.

Another potential source of exposure to radiation are whole-body CT scans, which some people are now requesting as part of a regular health checkup as a way to screen for cancer and other diseases. Many groups, including the FDA, have expressed concern over this practice because there is little evidence of its usefulness, and it exposes people to unnecessary radiation.

"Sometimes CT scans are available in shopping malls," says Boice. "They are advertising for healthy people to come in and get whole-body scans. This is unnecessary and inappropriate," he warns.

Whole-body CT scans do have their place. They can save the lives of accident victims who need quick evaluation to determine if they have a ruptured spleen or punctured lung. They are also effective in diagnosing some chronic conditions.

"The issue here is that one needs to be concerned about multiple CT scans," says Boice. "If you go to one hospital and have a CT scan and then go to another one and they do a follow-up, you should always question whether there is a need to do another CT scan. If you don't bring it to their attention, they may not know that CT scans or other x-rays have already been done. The bottom line is to ask the doctor if it is really necessary and to avoid, when possible, duplicate examinations."

Other Imaging Tests

Nuclear medicine tests, such as *positron emission tomography (PET)* scans, inject radioactive chemicals into the body. The amount of radiation used is quite small and is not considered a cancer risk. *Magnetic resonance imaging (MRI)* scanners, which rely on magnets, and *ultrasound* tests, which use sound waves, do not use radiation at all.

Knowing Your Environmental Risks

Unlike cancers caused by personal choices, some cancer risks are out of our control. There certainly must also be cancer-causing materials in our environment we don't even know about yet. But the good news is that we know a lot about what causes cancer in the world around us, and overall, the risks are small and generally avoidable.

In the next chapter, we'll look at cancer risks you might be exposed to in two specific environments—your home and your workplace.

CHAPTER 6

Dangers at Home and on the Job

D OCTORS IN NEBRASKA don't see many patients with cancer caused by asbestos, a group of naturally occurring fibrous minerals that are resistant to heat, making them popular for use as insulation and building materials. Doctors in East Coast cities, where asbestos was used in heavy manufacturing and shipbuilding, tend to see more such cases. So at first, none of the cancer specialists at the University of Nebraska Medical Center in Omaha suspected asbestos-related cancer in a tiny 73-year-old grandmother.

But when Myrna Block sought their opinion in 2001, all signs pointed to a very rare cancer called mesothelioma that affects the thin membranes lining the abdomen and chest. Exploratory surgery confirmed this most unusual and surprising diagnosis, and that's when the detective work began.

Where had she grown up? Lived? Worked? She had been a school-teacher and her husband an industrial engineer. They had been living with their three young children in Buffalo, New York, until his job brought them from the East Coast to Omaha in the 1970s. None of the puzzle pieces seemed to fit until doctors discovered that her husband's occupation, not hers, might have been the cause for her cancer. She revealed that her husband had worked at a company that used asbestos as lining for industrial fittings in the 1960s—more than 35 years ago.

Bingo! He carried home the tiny fibers on his clothing and body and in his hair. Because she had close contact with him and washed his clothes, she was exposed almost as intimately to the cancer-causing asbestos as if she herself had worked at the plant. The fibers had lain dormant in her body for decades, only to trigger one of the rarest and deadliest forms of cancer caused by an outside substance.

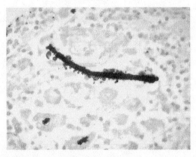

A microscopic view of lung tissue shows a fiber of asbestos. Image courtesy of Dr. Edwin P. Ewing, Jr., and the Centers for Disease Control and Prevention.

Most cases of mesothelioma result from asbestos exposure. According to the International Association for Research on Cancer (IARC), mesotheliomas have been observed not only among occupationally exposed workers but also among their family members, and people living in the neighborhoods surrounding asbestos factories and mines. Myrna Block's situation is not so unusual: a third of the mesothelioma cases in the United States may be due to such nonoccupational exposures.

Asbestos exposure can occur in your home or workplace. In this chapter, we'll consider cancer risks like asbestos that you may be exposed to at home or on the job.

Home Safe Home

Some controversial but unproven causes of cancer have gotten a lot of attention over the years. Valid concerns about cancer risk have focused a lot of attention on the products we use every day in our homes. But the results of isolated studies and misunderstandings about cause and effect have built up a frenzy about some factors in our homes that aren't cancer causing. So are antiperspirants linked to breast cancer? Will forgetting to wash an apple before eating it cause cancer? No, and no. Below are more details about common concerns about cancer and household items.

Eat, Drink, and Be Wary?

Food safety—specifically regarding pesticides and irradiation—has continued to be an issue of public concern in recent years. The majority of available scientific data, however, does not provide strong evidence for associations with cancer.

Plants, including many edible ones, naturally produce pesticides to protect themselves against insects. Some of these have been found to cause cancer in laboratory animals, but epidemiological studies have consistently found that a diet high in foods from plant sources is associated with a lower, rather than higher, risk of cancer.

Food Irradiation

Food irradiation has been used for decades to prevent illness caused by bacteria like *E. coli*, campylobacter, and salmonella and parasites in food, and sometimes irradiation is even used instead of pesticides. There is no credible evidence that irradiated foods cause cancer or that irradiation significantly affects the antioxidant vitamins and other substances in certain foods that may help prevent cancer.

Irradiation has been shown to be safe and effective, and it is now used in more than 40 countries. In the United States, the Food and Drug Administration (FDA) has approved the use of irradiation of meat and poultry and allows its use in some other foods as well, including fresh fruits and vegetables and spices.

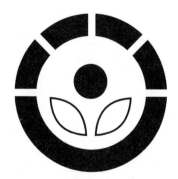

The FDA requires that irradiated foods include labeling with either the statement "treated with radiation" or "treated by irradiation" and the international symbol for irradiation, the radura.

In addition to reducing insects and parasites, irradiating certain fruits and vegetables delays ripening, allowing foods to remain unspoiled much longer. Irradiated strawberries, for example, stay unspoiled for up to three weeks. Untreated strawberries may last only three to five days.

The irradiation process exposes food to high frequency radiation (gamma rays or x rays) to kill the bacteria, but it does not make the food radioactive (just as an airport luggage scanner does not make luggage radioactive) or create harmful chemical compounds. It may cause a small loss of nutrients, but no more so than with other processing methods such as cooking, canning, or heat pasteurization.

Arsenic

A naturally occurring element in rocks and soil, *arsenic* can also be a byproduct of some industrial processes, and it was once a component of many pesticides. It has the potential to seep into underground water sources.

Capable of killing quickly in high doses, arsenic is a favorite poison in fictional crime stories like the classic black comedy *Arsenic and Old Lace*. But it can also prove fatal in very low doses when consumed over many years. A 1999 National Academy of Sciences report associated low levels of arsenic with bladder, lung, skin, and other cancers. Exposure may also lead to cardiovascular, immune system, nervous system, and hormonal diseases.

According to an article in the *New York Times*, 14 July 2002, millions of villagers in the country of Bangladesh rely on water from tube wells that tap into the region's underground aquifers, where arsenic occurs naturally. Unfortunately, the underground water sources were not tested for arsenic before the wells were set up. But affordable alternate water sources are not available to this very poor population.

Millions of Bangladeshis—about 26 percent of the population—drink arsenic-contaminated water on a daily basis, allowing the known human carcinogen to build up in their bodies over years. The World Health Organization (WHO) has called the situation "the largest mass poisoning of a population in history."

Allan H. Smith, M.D. and Ph.D., an epidemiologist at the University of California at Berkeley and an expert on arsenic, told the *New York Times* that the situation in Bangladesh is "the highest environmental cancer risk ever found."

These kinds of extreme cases of unsafe water are largely confined to developing countries without the resources to monitor and treat their water supplies. But arsenic is also a concern on a far lesser scale in some developed countries, including the United States.

Water in some areas of the United States, especially in Western states, contains arsenic, with the highest areas in the 50 to 100 parts per billion (ppb) range. (Compare this to Bangladesh, where the arsenic levels can be as high as several thousand ppb.) Most of the U.S. sites with high arsenic levels in drinking water are in rural communities and in places with private wells, including areas in the Southwest, Midwest, and New England. A few major cities, however, have higher-than-average levels of arsenic in the drinking water.

Recently, even "safe" levels of arsenic have been questioned. A report by the National Academy of Sciences (NAS) released in 2001 claims that arsenic in drinking water may be much more harmful than previously thought. Even tiny amounts of arsenic appear to be linked to increases in lung and bladder cancer. In fact, the EPA is reducing the amount of arsenic allowed in U.S. water supplies. This is a return to a tighter standard and will become fully effective in 2006.

The new standards will allow 10 parts per billion (ppb) of arsenic in drinking water for 74,000 water systems serving cities, towns, apartments, mobile home parks, schools, churches, nursing homes, factories, and other populations across the United States. Fifty parts per billion were allowed under the old rules.

The EPA expects the new standards to prevent up to 31 new cases of bladder cancer and 8 deaths from the disease each year, as well as 25 new cases of lung cancer and 22 deaths from lung cancer.

"The old standards were out of date and needed to be revised," concedes Jim Taft, chief of the Targeting and Analysis Branch of the EPA's Office of Ground Water and Drinking Water. "Arsenic is fairly widespread in the environment, but it tends primarily to be a ground water problem."

What's on Tap?

The Environmental Protection Agency (EPA) is responsible for assuring the safety of drinking water. It does this by setting drinking water standards—regulations to control the level of contaminants in the water. After reviewing studies that look at possible health effects, the EPA sets a maximum level of a contaminant in drinking water—a level that produces no expected effect on health and that also allows for a margin of safety.

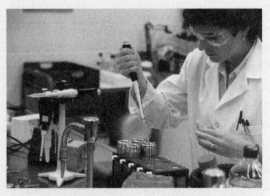

A scientist tests water samples for contaminants. Photo courtesy of the United States Environmental Protection Agency.

To address public concerns, in 1999 the EPA began requiring water suppliers to provide consumers with annual drinking water quality reports. Each July, you should receive a consumer confidence report from your water supplier in the mail, providing a summary of the susceptibility to contamination of the local drinking water source and information on nitrate, arsenic, or lead in areas where these contaminants are detected above 50 percent of the EPA standard.

The EPA has a local drinking water information web page (*http://epa.gov/safewater/dwinfo.htm*) that provides links to Internet-accessible water quality reports. For more information, you can call the EPA's Safe Drinking Water Hotline at 800-426-4791.

Pesticides on Food

Continued research is essential for maximum food safety, but pesticides play a valuable role in sustaining the food supply. In contrast to occupational and environmental health hazards, pesticide residues in the fruits and vegetables you buy or grow pose little to no risk to human health. In fact, people who eat more fruits and vegetables, which may have pesticide residues on them, generally have lower cancer risks than people who eat few fruits and vegetables.

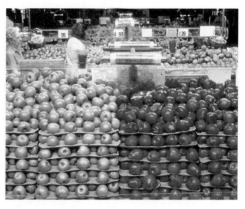

Apples purchased at the grocery store pose little to no risk of dangerous pesticide ingestion for consumers. Photo courtesy of Bill Branson and the National Cancer Institute.

The benefits of a balanced diet rich in fruits and vegetables far outweigh the largely theoretical risks posed by occasional, very low pesticide residue levels in foods.

If you are still concerned about pesticide residue on your fruits and vegetables, you can reduce and often eliminate residues present on food by following these tips provided by the FDA:

- Wash produce with large amounts of cold or warm tap water and scrub with a brush when appropriate. Do not use soap.

- Throw away the outer leaves of leafy vegetables such as lettuce and cabbage.

- Trim the fat from meat, and trim fat and skin from poultry and fish. (Residues of some pesticides concentrate in animal fat.)

You can also buy produce grown without manmade pesticides. These products are commonly labeled as "organically grown."

Artificial Sweeteners

For many years controversy has surrounded two approved sugar substitutes, saccharin and aspartame.

Discovered in 1879, saccharin is actually older than the FDA. When a Canadian study in the late 1970s showed that saccharin caused bladder cancer in rats, the FDA proposed to ban it. Because it was the only sugar substitute available at the time, a public outcry ensued, fueled in part by media reports that the test animals received the equivalent of hundreds of cans of diet soda a day. Congress responded by passing the Saccharin Study and Labeling Act, which placed a two-year moratorium on any ban of the sweetener while additional safety studies were conducted. The law required that any foods or beverages containing saccharin carry the warning: "Use of this product may be hazardous to your health. This product contains saccharin, which has been determined to cause cancer in laboratory animals."

Congress extended the moratorium several times, but recently gave saccharin a clean bill of health. Following the lead of the National Toxicology Program (NTP), who removed saccharin from its roster of "reasonably anticipated carcinogens" in 2000, Congress passed the so-called "SWEETEST" (Saccharin Warning Elimination via Environmental Testing Employing Science and Technology) Act repealing the law requiring warning labels on saccharin-sweetened foods.

Saccharin has remained on the market and continues to be in demand as a tabletop sweetener. It also has continuing appeal because of its long shelf life; because it is inexpensive to produce; and because of its stability at high temperatures (in contrast, aspartame is unstable at high temperatures, making it difficult to use as a sugar substitute in baked goods).

The bottom line: Studies have found that high doses of saccharin cause or promote tumors of the bladder in laboratory rodents. A closer look at the results of these rodent studies suggests they may not be relevant to humans. Because of differences in our metabolism, saccharin does not have the same effects on humans as on rats. Large epidemiological studies have not reported increased bladder cancers among people using saccharin; if saccharin does increase cancer risk in humans, it does so only at unusually high doses.

The FDA approved aspartame for use in 1981. It has been a controversial product ever since. Rumors of aspartame causing health problems have abounded, linking it to everything from autoimmune diseases, such as lupus and multiple sclerosis, to brain cancer. But there is very little, if any, evidence to back up any of these claims—other than the known risk to people with a rare genetic defect known as *phenylketonuria* (a disorder in which people cannot metabolize the naturally occurring amino acid phenylalanine, a chemical found in aspartame.)

Aflatoxin

Not all cancer-causing substances are manmade. The most well-known "natural" carcinogen is *aflatoxin*, a chemical produced by mold that sometimes contaminates peanuts, wheat, soybeans, ground nuts, corn, and rice. Aflatoxin causes liver cancer and contributes significantly to that disease in parts of Africa, where food spoilage caused by molds is common. In the United States, there is a comprehensive program that requires the USDA and FDA to test certain foods to ensure that they do not contain dangerous amounts of aflatoxin. Peanuts and peanut products are among the most stringently tested, so the risk of developing liver cancer from your peanut butter and jelly sandwich is remote!

Peanuts are stringently tested for the presence of aflatoxin, a cancer-causing agent. Photos courtesy of Renee Comet and the National Cancer Institute.

Personal Products

Personal care products like cosmetics, hair and skin care items, fragrances, toothpastes, and deodorants have been used for centuries. Should you be concerned about potential dangers in your medicine cabinet? Many of the purported risks shared through e-mails are not carcinogens. But some personal products may put you at increased risk for cancer.

Hair Dye

About one-third of adult American women, as well as a small but increasing number of men, use hair dyes. Hair color is important to many people, but does it cause cancer?

Most of the concern about potential cancer risk revolves around the use of permanent and semi-permanent dyes, as opposed to temporary ones (those lasting only a few washings). These products contain chemicals that have been found to cause cancer in laboratory animals. The animals in these studies, however, were fed high levels of the dyes over a long period of time, so the relevance of this information to the use of hair dyes by humans is uncertain. Because dark brown and black dyes have higher concentrations of suspected carcinogens, these products are of greatest potential concern.

More than 20 studies across large populations have examined the association between exposure to permanent hair dyes and various cancers. The largest studies to date have found that death rates from all cancers combined appear to be about the same for women who use hair dyes and those who do not. Some studies have found an association between hair dye use and bladder or blood cancers (such as leukemias), but others have not.

Most hair dyes don't have to go through the safety testing that other cosmetic color additives do before hitting store shelves. But most available evidence does not show hair dyes to be a significant cancer risk factor.

So what if you regularly dye your hair? Other than recommendations that apply to everyone when it comes to routine health screening and healthy lifestyle choice, no specific medical advice is needed for current or former hair dye users. The bottom line is that most of the available evidence does not show hair dyes to be a significant cancer risk factor.

If you are still concerned about even potential risks, the FDA suggests you do the following:

- Don't leave the dye on your head any longer than necessary.

- Rinse your scalp thoroughly with water after use.

- Wear gloves when applying hair dye.

- Carefully follow the directions.

- Never mix different hair-dye products, because you can induce potentially harmful reactions.

- If you haven't used a dye before, be sure to do a patch test for allergic reactions before applying the dye to your hair.

- Never dye your eyebrows or eyelashes.

- Delay dyeing your hair until later in life when it starts to turn gray.

- Consider using henna (largely plant-derived), hair dyes that are lead acetate-based, or temporary hair coloring products. These colorings don't fall into the coal-tar dye category and therefore any additive ingredients they contain have been tested for safety before marketing, in accordance with FDA requirements.

Talc

Talc, also known as talcum powder, is a white to grayish white powder. It is found in most body and baby powders, except those that are specifically labeled "talc-free" or "pure cornstarch" and is also used for medicinal and toiletry products, glove and shoe powders, fillers for pills, and soap and paper products.

Talc may be contaminated with other minerals like asbestos, silica, or quartz. Several studies have examined the connection between talc inhalation exposure among certain workers and lung cancer. In many of the studies with positive results, there was evidence of asbestos contamination of the talc. In these cases, the substance responsible for the cancers may have been asbestos rather than the talc. Thus, the evidence for lung cancer is strongest for talc contaminated by asbestos. There is little available evidence to suggest that the grade of talc now used in consumer products increases the risk of developing lung cancer.

Several studies in the 1980s and 1990s suggested that the use of talc in genital hygiene products could lead to the development of ovarian cancer. Again, this link may be due to the presence of asbestos fibers in talc, because the two substances are often found together in mineral deposits. There is a need for further research on this link.

Neither the NTP nor the EPA has classified talc as carcinogenic. However, talc that contains asbestos is known to be carcinogenic. The IARC does not have enough evidence to classify talc not containing asbestos as carcinogenic.

Nonetheless, if you are concerned about the use of talc or genital powders, you may wish to reduce your use of powders or use only cornstarch powders. A recent review suggests that cornstarch is unlikely to increase cancer risk.

Antiperspirants

There is no scientific evidence to support the much-hyped link between antiperspirants and breast cancer, according to a recent study. This rumor circulated so widely on the Internet it became a public concern, a kind of urban myth, despite the fact there had not been any published, scientific reports suggesting any such association.

The widely circulated theory that nicks from razors supposedly allow antiperspirants to be absorbed into the body, preventing the lymph nodes under the arms from removing cancer-causing toxins from the breasts, is not valid.

No population-based studies have reported an association between breast cancer risk and antiperspirant use. There is also no evidence that the chemicals in antiperspirants are absorbed through the skin (regardless of whether the skin is shaved or has small razor nicks). There is also no evidence that aluminum or any of the other chemicals found in antiperspirants cause DNA damage that can lead to cancer.

Sweat glands, located in the skin, are not connected to lymph nodes. Lymph nodes help clear some potentially cancer-causing toxins from the body, but they do not release these toxins through sweating. The fluid in lymph nodes enters the bloodstream, where toxins are eventually removed by the liver (and excreted in feces) or kidneys (and excreted in urine).

Some women may wonder why they are advised not to use antiperspirants or deodorants on the day they are scheduled to receive a mammogram. Here's why: many of these products contain aluminum, a metal that can show up on a mammogram as tiny specks. These specks can resemble microcalcifications, one of the things doctors look for as a possible sign of cancer. Avoiding the use of these products helps prevent any confusion when looking at the mammogram films.

Cleaning Products

By their very nature, many chemicals used in cleaning products have toxic properties like being poisonous or corrosive. Does this mean we should avoid using them to scrub our toilets or unclog our drains? Not at all! When used properly, most of them pose little or no health risk. What's important is not the *potential* of the substance to do harm, but the actual risk to *you* in how you use the product. When it comes to cancer risk, most household cleaners are reasonably safe. They are more likely to pose an immediate threat as a poison or a corrosive, so it is especially important to store them away from where children can reach them.

What to Do When You Have Questions About a Specific Product

A certain amount of safety information should be available on a product's label. If not, you can find out more from the National Institute of Environmental Health Sciences (NIEHS) Office of Communications at (919) 541-3345 (*www.niehs.nih.gov/external/faq/hsprod.htm*).

For specific information about possible carcinogenic properties, you may also want to visit the Web site of the International Agency for Research on Cancer (IARC) (*http://monographs.iarc.fr/*) or the United States National Toxicology Program NTP (*http://ntp-server.niehs.nih.gov/*) to look for the product's ingredients on the complete lists of carcinogenic agents.

Household Pesticides

According to the EPA's Office of Pesticide Programs, a *pesticide* is any substance or mixture of substances intended for preventing, destroying, repelling, or reducing any pest. Pests can be insects, mice, and other animals, unwanted plants (weeds), fungi, or microorganisms like bacteria and viruses. Though often misunderstood to refer only to *insecticides*, the term pesticide also applies to *herbicides* and *fungicides*.

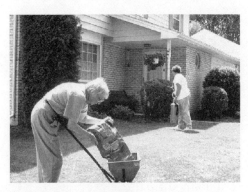

The health risks of pesticides are primarily from direct contact with chemicals at high doses. Photo courtesy of the United States Geological Survey, *http://water.usgs.gov/pubs/circ/circ1158/circ1158.pdf.*

About 75 percent of homes in the United States use at least one pesticide product indoors each year. In fact, most household exposure to pesticides occurs inside the home rather than outside. The sources include airborne particles, chemicals tracked in from outdoors, and stored pesticide containers.

But the health hazards of pesticides are primarily from direct contact with the chemicals at high doses. For example, at great risk are farm workers who apply the chemicals and work in the fields after the pesticides have been applied, and people living near fields sprayed from the air.

The health effects most often associated with high-dose pesticide exposure include irritation to the eyes, nose, and throat, dizziness, muscle twitching, tingling sensations, and nausea. Repeated and long-term exposure can ultimately cause damage to the central nervous system, liver, and kidneys, and, for some pesticides, an increased risk of cancer.

Pesticides and Breast Cancer

In recent years, some controversy has existed around the possible relationship between certain pesticides and cancers that are influenced by hormones, such as breast cancer. *Dichloro-diphenyl-trichloroethane (DDT)* and other organochlorine insecticides have been implicated because of their ability to mimic the effects of estrogen, a major female hormone. Although DDT and some of the organochlorine insecticides were banned from use in the United States in the 1970s, questions about their lingering effects remain.

Currently, research does not show a clear link between breast cancer risk and exposure to these environmental pollutants. Although a few studies have suggested certain pollutants increase breast cancer risk, the most recent analysis of available data, combining the results from several previous studies of women living in the northeastern United States, did not find such a link. Most experts believe that if such a connection exists, it accounts for only a few breast cancer cases, but research in this area continues.

Herbicides and Lymphoma

Herbicides are chemicals that kill plants—weeds in particular. There are many chemical classes of herbicides, but it is the *phenoxy herbicides* (such as 2,4-dichlorophenoxyacetic acid, 2,4-D for short, and 2,4,5-trichlorophenoxyacetic acid, 2,4,5-T for short) that have been of greatest concern as a possible carcinogen.

Several studies have suggested an increased risk of non-Hodgkin's lymphoma among farmers, and herbicides were one of the possible explanations considered. Those studies are limited by absence of dose information, mixed chemical exposures, and exposures to infections and other possible causes of cancer. More recent epidemiologic studies have focused on herbicide industry workers. These have suggested a possible trend toward slightly increased risk of non-Hodgkin's lymphoma in relation to phenoxy herbicide exposure. But the results have been inconsistent and the association, if present, appears to be weak. Animal evidence has not shown the phenoxy herbicides to be carcinogenic. Most expert agencies have found that no firm conclusions can be drawn.

Dangerous Work

About 20,000 cancer deaths and 40,000 new cases of cancer each year in the United States are attributable to occupation, according to the National Institute for Occupational Safety and Health (NIOSH), the federal agency responsible for conducting research and making recommendations to prevent work-related disease and energy.

"Millions of U.S. workers are exposed to substances that have tested as carcinogens in animal studies," NIOSH warns on its Web site. (These results do not definitively prove that these substances cause cancer in humans.) It adds that fewer than two percent of chemicals currently in use by commerce have been tested for carcinogenicity.

Some industries dealing with substances that potentially contribute to cancer include the following:

- aluminum production

- boot and shoe manufacture and repair

- furniture and cabinet making

- hematite mining (underground) with exposure to radon

- iron and steel founding

- nickel refining

- nuclear weapons industry

- painting (occupational exposure)

- rubber industry

Nuclear Fallout

During the Cold War, the United States' nuclear weapons industry employed 200,000 people. Hundreds of thousands of others worked for the industry in support jobs.

Who's on the Job?

Although NIOSH and OSHA were both created by the Occupational Safety and Health Act of 1970, they are two distinct agencies with separate responsibilities. NIOSH is a research agency and part of the Centers for Disease Control and Prevention (CDC), while OSHA is a regulatory agency and part of the Department of Labor (DOL). OSHA is responsible for creating and enforcing workplace safety and health regulations. You can contact either of these agencies if you have questions or concerns about hazards in your workplace.

"They worked with the most dangerous chemicals ever invented, under conditions of great secrecy. Their primary mission was to build nuclear weapons, and safety often took a back seat," says David Michaels, Ph.D., M.P.H., a research professor in the Department of Environmental and Occupational Health at George Washington University in Washington, D.C.

Technicians handling radioactive plutonium wore protective gear and worked with special glove boxes that occasionally leaked, exposing them to radiation. Other workers were charged with tasks like running machines to shape beryllium—a metal now known to cause lung cancer—into nuclear weapons components. "In some cases they wore masks," Michaels explains, "But we now know that many types of respirators are not effective for blocking out beryllium [dust]."

Michaels, who served as the U.S. Department of Energy Assistant Secretary for Environment, Safety and

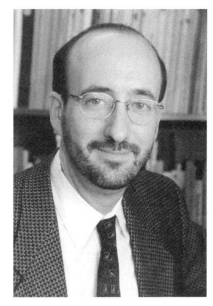

David Michaels, Ph.D., M.P.H.

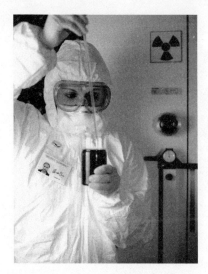

Many government workers developed cancer or lung disease after exposure to materials used in the making of nuclear weapons.

Health from 1998 to 2001, worked for years to gain compensation for workers in the nuclear weapons complex who developed cancer or lung disease after exposure to radiation, beryllium, and other hazards.

The historic Energy Employee Occupational Illness Compensation Program Act was passed in 2000; in its first 2 years the program awarded more than 400 million dollars in benefits to workers with cancer or lung disease. Improved technologies and tighter regulations have made those working with nuclear materials much safer than during the Cold War.

Working with Asbestos

Asbestos is used to insulate buildings and pipes and to make car brake and clutch parts, roofing shingles, ceiling and floor tiles, cement, textiles, and hundreds of other products. Inhaling asbestos fibers has been proven to cause pulmonary cancers.

People are exposed to asbestos mainly through inhalation of fibers in the air they breathe. Those with the heaviest exposure worked in asbestos industries like shipbuilding and insulating. People can also be exposed when older asbestos-containing materials begin to break down.

"There is no question that the environmental protections in place today are far better than those of 30 years ago," Michaels observes. "Certainly we are doing better on asbestos and some other well-known carcinogens. Most of the lawsuits [filed by workers over asbestos-related illnesses] are from decades-old exposures." But there is much room for improvement, he adds.

Although the risk of asbestos exposure has dropped dramatically in the United States, there is still a potential for exposure from asbestos that remains in older buildings, around water pipes, and in other settings. If there is a possibility of on-the-job exposure, use the protective equipment, work practices, and safety procedures designed for working around asbestos. If you live in an older home and have damaged insulation, have an expert check to find out if there is any asbestos and if it poses any risk of exposure. Asbestos is not always an immediate hazard. It causes problems when it is disturbed. Some experts may recommend leaving it alone and periodically checking it. If it's a significant risk, you may need to have an experienced contractor remove any asbestos in your home.

Exposure to Benzene

Benzene is a colorless, flammable liquid with a sweet odor that forms from natural processes, like volcanic eruptions and forest fires, and from human activities, such as smoking. (Benzene is a component of cigarette smoke.) Benzene is also manufactured and widely used in the United States as a solvent (used to dissolve substances), a starting material for combining other chemicals, and in gasoline.

The greatest risk for exposure to high doses of benzene is in industries that make or use benzene. But benzene also exists in low levels in the environment and in some cleaning products.

Both the IARC and the NTP classify benzene as a known human carcinogen. The evidence linking benzene and cancer comes mainly from studying workers in the chemical, shoemaking, and oil refining industries that developed acute myelogenous leukemia (AML), a cancer of blood-forming cells in the bone marrow.

EPA regulation restricts concentrations of benzene in drinking water to five parts per billion, with an ultimate goal of zero parts per billion. NIOSH and OSHA have limited acceptable occupational exposures to benzene to 0.1 parts per million and also recommend personal protective equipment like respirators when working with this substance.

Other Workers at Risk

Certain cancers have been linked to carpentry and furniture making and refinishing. Since the 1960s, researchers have noticed higher rates of cancer of the nose, voice box (larynx), and lungs in people who work in the furniture manufacturing industry. The IARC has since determined that exposure to hardwood dust increases the risk for

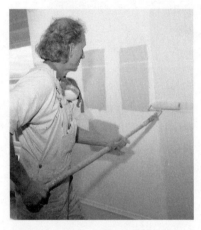

these types of cancer. Woodworkers (even in home workshops) should wear masks and use suction or vacuum devices for equipment that creates sawdust.

As mentioned earlier, workers exposed to high levels of pesticides in industry or farming may be at higher risk of certain cancers. Another occupation that has raised some questions about cancer risk is painting. As a group, painters show an increased incidence of lung cancer, possibly due to exposure to *methylene chloride*

Individuals in certain occupations may be at higher risk for some cancers. For example, painters are at greater risk for lung cancer.

(used as a solvent or paint remover) and the glycol ethers in paints.

Living Safely

Sometimes environmental factors—some we can closely control and others we can't—play a role, directly or indirectly, in cancer cases. Should we live in a bubble or spend all of our time worrying about potential discoveries of new cancer-causing materials? Of course not.

Unfortunately there are many aspects of cancer and what causes it that the scientific community hasn't yet proven. But through population-based studies and laboratory experiments, we can get a reasonable idea of many associations between exposures in the home and at work and the development of cancer. Being aware of established risks and knowing the rumors about carcinogens will help you both protect your health and keep fears in check.

CHAPTER 7

The Keys Are in Our Hands

B RITISH CANCER RESEARCHER SIR RICHARD DOLL, M.D., started smoking in 1931, when he was 19 years old. "My father, a general practitioner, offered me 50 pounds—which was a lot of money in those days—if I didn't start smoking until I was 21," Doll recalls. "The reason he did that wasn't because he thought that smoking was bad for you. He thought it was a waste of money."

The teenaged Doll was determined to get the payoff from his father and held off smoking for a while, even though most of his friends had started the habit.

"I had an irritating little brother, seven years younger than me, who used to pipe up at parties and say, 'Richard can't smoke until he's 21 because then he'll get 50 pounds,'" Doll says. "So one day when he did that I just said, 'Oh, for God's sake! I can't stand it, give me a cigarette.'"

With that gesture, Doll joined the ranks of 80 percent of British males who smoked regularly during that era. Smoking was so prevalent that some physicians used to offer their patients a cigarette to put them at ease when they came in for consultations.

"It was just a normal part of life that one didn't question," Doll recalls.

In 1947, Doll became part of a team assigned by the British Medical Research Council to determine why the incidence of lung cancer had gone up rapidly since the beginning of the 1900s.

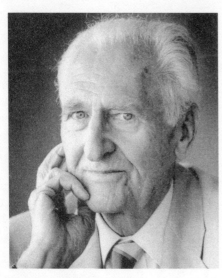

Sir Richard Doll, M.D.

The evidence was clear and convincing to Doll, who stubbed out his last cigarette in 1949, as the study results accumulated. In their quest for more decisive evidence that smoking causes lung cancer, Doll and his colleague, Sir Austin Bradford Hill, sent questionnaires to thousands of British doctors in 1951, asking about their health and smoking habits. Ultimately, 40,000 physicians agreed to take part in a long-term study.

"Within five years we were finding that many of those who smoked heavily got lung cancer and the ones who didn't smoke didn't get it," Doll says. But it took many more years before society at large could be convinced of the dangers of tobacco.

The study of the smoking habits of British doctors continued until 2001. "We were discovering new things for quite a long time," Doll says. "When we started, we wanted to predict who would get lung cancer. By the time we got clear data for lung cancer, we were finding increases for myocardial infarction [in smokers]. We went on getting more information about different diseases for many years. We found that the effects of smoking in the last 20 years of the study were greater than in the first 20 years, and that lifelong cigarette smoking is much more hazardous than had been appreciated."

Doll, now 90 years old, is the honorary consultant to Cancer Research U.K. and still goes to work each day at the Clinical Trial

Service Unit and Epidemiological Studies Unit at the Radcliffe Infirmary in Oxford, England.

Lifestyle: Multiple Choice

In the last two chapters, we discussed environmental causes of cancer that we're exposed to in a passive way. In this chapter, we'll explore environmental causes of cancer that are probably much more important: the choices people make every day and how those choices affect their health.

The way we live our lives determines a large part of our cancer risk. Lifestyle and other controllable risk factors are linked to over two-thirds of cancer deaths. Lifestyle factors that affect cancer risk include:

Tobacco: Tobacco smoke is one of the most studied carcinogens, and tobacco is associated with more than a dozen types of cancer. The proof that smoking can cause lung cancer—the leading cause of cancer death for both men and women in the United States—is overwhelming.

Nutrition: Decades of nutritional research shows that dietary choices are a factor in about one-third of fatal cancers.

Physical Activity: Research indicates that keeping physically active reduces the risk of some cancers.

Alcohol: Alcohol increases the risk of cancers of the mouth, pharynx, larynx, esophagus, liver, and breast. Regularly drinking even one alcoholic beverage a day is associated with an increased risk of breast cancer in women.

"We're talking close to 370,000 cancer deaths a year that could be prevented if people didn't smoke, ate well, and lived an active lifestyle," says Colleen Doyle, M.S., R.D., director of nutrition and physical activity for the American Cancer Society (ACS). That number is much higher when the deaths from heart disease, stroke, emphysema, diabetes, and other chronic diseases that are related to smoking, diet, and weight are factored in.

You probably already know that food, exercise, tobacco, and alcohol affect your health. We're not here to preach about what you *should* do—you'll make your own choices. But since this is a book about what causes cancer, it's only fitting that we get into the science of how and why these lifestyle factors affect your cancer risk.

Tobacco Use: The Nation's Leading Cause of Death

According to the Centers for Disease Control and Prevention, each year approximately 406, 290 people in the United States die as a result of smoking cigarettes*. The majority of these smoking-related deaths are from lung cancer, but smoking-related deaths are also caused by coronary heart disease, chronic lung disease, other diagnoses, other cancers, and stroke.

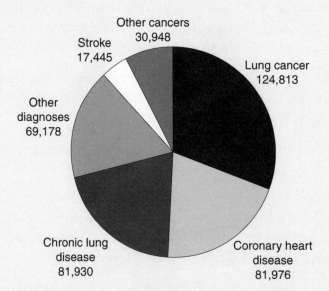

*Average annual number of deaths, 1995-1999
Source: CDC. Annual smoking-attributable mortality, years of potential life lost, and economic costs—United States—1995-1999. *MMWR* 2002;51(14):300–3.

Tobacco Timeline

Tobacco has been around for hundreds of years. Native Americans revered tobacco for its "medicinal" and ceremonial uses. Christopher Columbus brought tobacco back to Spain from the Americas, and by the mid-sixteenth century people began to smoke in Europe. By 1612, Englishman John Rolfe had begun the first tobacco plantation in Virginia, and tobacco soon became the colony's biggest crop.

Tobacco smoke was a suspected carcinogen as early as the eighteenth century, but it wasn't until 1930 that researchers in Cologne, Germany, made a statistical correlation between cancer and smoking. In 1938, Raymond Pearl, Ph.D., of Johns Hopkins University in Baltimore, Maryland, reported in *Science* magazine that smokers do not live as long as nonsmokers.

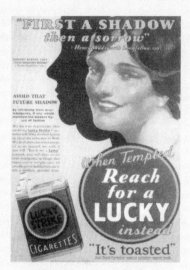

By 1944 the ACS warned consumers that smoking might have negative health effects, although it had no definite evidence. In 1952, *Reader's Digest* published "Cancer by the Carton," which outlined the dangers of smoking. Other publications began printing similar articles, and some smokers began to become wary of smoking.

Early advertisements for tobacco did not warn users of its dangerous health effects. Ad courtesy of Virginia Ernster, Ph.D.

In 1964, on the basis of more than 7,000 articles relating to smoking and disease available at that time in biomedical literature, the Surgeon General's Advisory Committee concluded that cigarette smoking is a cause of lung cancer and laryngeal cancer in men, a probable cause of lung cancer in women, and the most important cause of chronic bronchitis.

Lung cancer was a rare form of cancer until the twentieth century. As more and more people were sold on cigarettes, lung cancer changed from an uncommon affliction into a national plague. Today, lung cancer is the leading cause of cancer death for both men and women in the United States.

The Smoking Gun: Tobacco

Everyone knows that tobacco and its smoke are major causes of cancer. But smoking is addictive, and many people smoke even though they know it's not a good health choice. Most smokers start the habit as impressionable teenagers, and when they become adults they find it extremely difficult to stop smoking. Smoking is highly addictive—nicotine's addictiveness is often compared to that of cocaine or heroin—and quitting can be extremely difficult for those who become hooked. About 70 percent of smokers say they would like to quit.

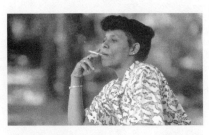

Approximately 23 percent of the U.S. population regularly smokes cigarettes. Photo courtesy of Bill Branson and the National Cancer Institute.

Yet almost one in four American adults still smokes despite overwhelming evidence of the risks. Smoking-related diseases claim over 400,000 American lives each year. Smoking costs the United States approximately $97.2 billion each year in health-care costs and lost productivity. It is responsible for 87 percent of lung cancer cases.

The Face of Smokers

According to the Centers for Disease Control and Prevention, as of the year 2000, an estimated 46.5 million adults were current smokers—about 23 percent of the population in the United States.

- **Gender:** The prevalence of smoking was higher among men (25.7%) than women (21.0%).

- **Race and Ethnicity:** Asians (14.4%) and Hispanics (18.6%) had the lowest prevalence of adult cigarette use; American Indians/Alaska Natives had the highest prevalence (36.0%).

- **Education Level:** Adults with a General Educational Development (GED) diploma had the highest prevalence

(47.2%) of smoking; persons with master's, professional, and doctoral degrees had the lowest prevalence (8.4%).

- **Socioeconomic Status:** The prevalence of current smoking was higher among adults living below the poverty level (31.7%) than among those at or above the poverty level (22.9%).

The New Face of Smokers: Youth

During the years 1993–2000, substantial reductions in current smoking prevalence were reported for all age groups, except 18–24 year olds. The vast majority of new customers for cigarettes come from the ranks of teenagers.

Nearly one-third of high school students are current smokers. More than 80 percent of adult tobacco users started their habit before they were 18 years old, according to the Department of Health and Human Services. According to the CDC, more than 6.4 million children living today will die prematurely because of a decision they will make as adolescents—the decision to start smoking.

A Worldwide Crisis

Smoking is an even a bigger problem internationally. According to the American Lung Association, 1.1 billion people—one-third of the global population aged 15 years and older—are regular smokers. Tobacco use kills four million people every year around the globe. The death toll is expected to go up to 8.4 million per year by 2020 and ten million annually in 2030. If the estimates are correct, the World Health Organization warns, tobacco will become the world's largest single health problem.

Tobacco control is a well-established concept in the developed world, but much of the developing world is either unaware of the dangers of tobacco or unable to fight the economic and political clout of international tobacco companies.

The Ugly Truth

Lung cancer kills more Americans each year than any other cancer. Lung cancer kills more people than breast, prostate, and colorectal cancers *combined*. It is hard to detect it in its earliest stage and is one of the most difficult cancers to treat.

Fewer than 15 percent of people with lung cancer live longer than five years.

Lung cancer is largely preventable. About 87 percent of lung cancer deaths are related to smoking.

Lung cancer is not the only cancer caused by smoking. Smoking is also linked with cancers of the mouth, throat, esophagus, pancreas, cervix, kidney, and bladder. Recent studies have indicated that smoking may also be associated with cancers of the stomach, liver, colon, and rectum, and with a form of acute leukemia as well.

The Anatomy of a Cigarette

"The public perception is that a cigarette is a natural product because tobacco is an organic plant material," says Jeffrey Wigand, Ph.D., former executive with Brown & Williamson, owned by BAT Industries, the world's second largest tobacco company. "But cigarettes are not a natural product at all. Think of them as highly sophisticated drug-delivery devices that deliver an addictive substance—nicotine—along with thousands of other toxins."

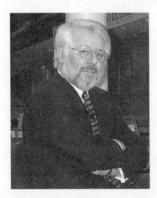

Jeffrey Wigand, Ph.D.

Wigand knows cigarettes from the inside out. An influential tobacco executive, he blew the whistle in 1995 on the industry's disregard for public health. The ensuing court battles became the subject of a movie, *The Insider*, and Wigand

You Are What You Smoke

Approximately 4,000 known chemical compounds are present in tobacco smoke. Here are a few of them.

- *nicotine*: a highly addictive and toxic substance that is the active ingredient in many insecticides
- *hydrogen cyanide*: a poisonous gas used to execute prisoners in gas chambers
- *formaldehyde*: a toxic gas used to preserve body tissue
- *ammonia*: a pungent, suffocating gas and a powerful agent used in cleaning
- *arsenic*: a potent poison
- *methanol*: a poisonous substance used for solvents, jet engine and rocket fuels, and in antifreeze
- *cadmium*: a metallic element, found in car batteries
- *butane*: a flammable chemical used for lighter fuel and in the manufacturing process of rubber
- *acetone*: a poisonous solvent used as a paint stripper and nail polish remover
- *toluene*: a poisonous industrial solvent, also used in the manufacture of TNT
- *polonium-210*: a highly radioactive element
- *carbon monoxide*: an odorless poisonous gas found in car exhaust
- *benzene*: a toxin derived from coal tar and used chiefly in the manufacture of dyes and as a solvent

went on to form Smoke-Free Kids, Inc., to educate children about the dangers of tobacco use.

The cigarette manufacturing process begins, Wigand explains, with tobacco leaves that naturally contain nicotine, a highly addictive substance that can also be poisonous. The leaves may also contain residues of pesticides used in the growing process and traces of substances that occur naturally in the soil, such as arsenic, radioactive polonium, chromium, as well as other heavy metals. During the curing process, carcinogenic byproducts called *nitrosamines* are formed. Later, in the manufacturing process, hundreds of chemicals are added to the cured tobacco.

So what is it about cigarettes that cause cancer? Matt Barry, M.P.A., a researcher for the Washington-based National Center for Tobacco-Free Kids, says that tobacco smoke is a "chemical soup." He notes that by 1989, researchers had found 43 carcinogens in tobacco smoke. By 2000, the National Cancer Institute reported that 69 carcinogens had been detected. "As the evidence base grows and people study these things in detail, the list keeps growing," Barry says.

Cigarettes are not the only culprit. There is no safe tobacco product. The use of *any* tobacco product—including cigars, pipes, smokeless or "spit" tobacco, and mentholated, "low-tar," "naturally grown," or "additive-free" tobacco—can cause cancer and other adverse health effects.

Defending Your Lungs

The human lungs have a remarkable design, but they are no match for the onslaught of chemicals in tobacco smoke, according to David Burns, M.D., a pulmonologist and professor of medicine at the University of California at San Diego School of Medicine.

Burns explains that the surface area of the lungs is nearly the size of a tennis court. It's folded over and over into tiny grapelike clusters called *alveoli*—between 300 million and 400 million in each lung. When you breathe in, the alveoli pull oxygen into the bloodstream, and push out unneeded carbon dioxide, which you then exhale.

Cigarette smoke, however, causes inflammation and irritation, which narrow the tubes in the lungs that people breathe through, making it more difficult to move air back and forth. It also breaks down the walls between the alveoli, making small alveoli into bigger ones and decreasing the surface area of the lungs so that they have less contact with oxygen.

Still, your lungs are remarkably resilient organs. "Many smokers believe if they have been smoking for years, the damage has been done and there is no use in trying to stop," says Ron Todd, M.S., Ed.D., director of tobacco control for the ACS. "But regardless of how many years you've smoked, quitting can still result in many health benefits. The body does a remarkable job of repairing itself. But the sooner you quit, the better."

Secondhand Smoke Stinks

Even if you have never smoked or quit smoking a long time ago, you may have health effects from smoking. "It is now clear that disease risk due to inhalation of tobacco smoke is not limited to the individual who is smoking," says C. Everett Koop, M.D., former U.S. Surgeon General. As an involuntary smoker—a nonsmoker breathing the smoke exhaled by others, as well as smoke from burning cigarettes themselves—you are at increased risk. Smoke from others is also called environmental tobacco smoke, *passive* or *involuntary smoking*, or secondhand smoke.

Your risk of developing disease depends on the amount of tobacco smoke to which you are exposed. An involuntary smoker inhales less tobacco smoke than an active smoker because the smoke mixes with the air around them. But the Environmental Protection Agency (EPA) estimates that secondhand smoke causes about 3,000 lung cancer deaths each year in nonsmoking adults and impairs the respiratory health of hundreds of thousands of children.

Exposure to cigar smoke is even worse. Secondhand smoke from cigars contains many of the same poisons and cancer-causing agents as cigarette smoke, but in higher concentrations and greater amounts, because cigars often burn longer and give off more smoke.

People who have smokers in their families have as much as a 30 percent higher chance of dying from lung cancer as those who live in a family of nonsmokers. Involuntary smoking also causes heart disease, aggravates asthma, and impairs blood circulation.

The Power of Diet and Exercise

For the majority of Americans who don't smoke, nutrition and physical activity are the most important cancer risk factors they can modify to reduce cancer risk. "Except for smoking, obesity is now the number one preventable cause of death in this country," says Koop.

During the past 20 years, studies have provided convincing evidence that a healthy diet and a healthy body weight are vital to lowering risks for many chronic diseases, including cancer. During the same 20-year period, Americans have grown progressively more overweight.

"When you look at the trends for those who are overweight, it's happening in all age groups and all races, across the board," notes Doyle. "It's an enormous problem that needs to be dealt with." She goes on to say that looking good isn't the only reason to eat healthy and exercise; paying attention to diet and physical activity can save lives. Eating a healthy diet and being physically active can help your health and affect cancer risk at any stage of life.

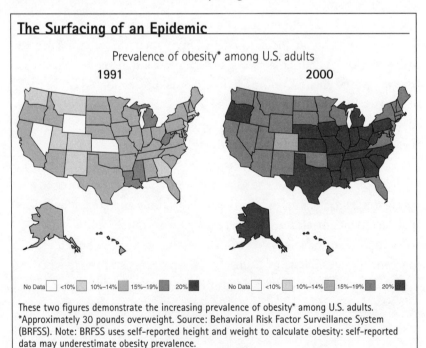

The Surfacing of an Epidemic

Prevalence of obesity* among U.S. adults

1991   **2000**

No Data ☐   <10% ☐   10%–14% ☐   15%–19% ☐   20% ☐

These two figures demonstrate the increasing prevalence of obesity* among U.S. adults. *Approximately 30 pounds overweight. Source: Behavioral Risk Factor Surveillance System (BRFSS). Note: BRFSS uses self-reported height and weight to calculate obesity: self-reported data may underestimate obesity prevalence.

American Cancer Society Diet and Exercise Guidelines for Cancer Prevention

No diet is guaranteed to provide full protection against any disease, but the ACS believes that the following guidelines offer the best nutrition and physical activity information currently available to help Americans reduce their risk of cancer.

1. Eat a variety of healthful foods, with an emphasis on plant sources.
- Eat five or more servings of a variety of vegetables and fruits each day. (A standard serving of most fruits and vegetables is one-half cup.)

- Choose whole grains over processed (refined) grains and sugars.

- Limit consumption of red meats, especially those high in fat and processed.

- Choose foods that help you maintain a healthful weight.

2. Adopt a physically active lifestyle.
- Adults: engage in at least moderate activity for 30 minutes or more on five or more days of the week; 45 minutes or more of moderate-to-vigorous activity on five or more days per week may further enhance reductions in the risk of breast and colon cancer.

- Children and adolescents: engage in at least 60 minutes per day of moderate-to-vigorous physical activity at least five days per week.

3. Maintain a healthful weight throughout life.
- Balance caloric intake with physical activity.

- Lose weight if currently overweight or obese.

4. If you drink alcoholic beverages, limit your consumption.

Today, more than 64 percent of adult Americans are overweight, and nearly 31 percent are obese. Even more alarming, obesity rates in children have more than doubled over the past two decades.

One factor that contributes to the problem is technological convenience, which cuts back on traditional expenditures of physical energy that were once considered routine. A lack of pedestrian-friendly areas and a tendency to lounge indoors in front of the television or computer also squelch activity. Americans—especially children—often eat large portions, including many foods that are not nutritional.

It can also be difficult to sort out all the conflicting information about hot new diets, "miracle" supplements, and the latest scientific findings for particular foods. That means that even when people take the time and effort to plan and prepare a healthy meal, they are sometimes unsure about what exactly they should be eating.

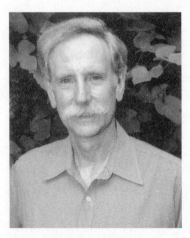

Walter Willett, M.D., Dr.P.H.

"There is a lot of confusion," says Walter Willett, M.D., Dr.P.H., chairman of the Department of Nutrition at the Harvard School of Public Health and a professor of medicine at Harvard Medical School. "People are given strong messages without a lot of data, and then new data comes along that may not support earlier beliefs. The public has a doubly hard time sorting this out because they often just get little bits and pieces of unconfirmed findings. It's pretty amazing that people are not more confused than they are."

A Balancing Act

The basic principles of healthy eating are actually rather simple: Eat a varied diet of primarily plant-based foods, limit your intake of saturated fats, and maintain a healthy weight. "When you look back on decades of research and recommendations of healthy eating, that's what always rings true," Doyle said. "It's all about balance."

Other key points to keep in mind when attempting to lower cancer risk are to:

- cut back on red meat, which is high in saturated fat

- choose whole grains over refined carbohydrates

- eat five or more servings of fruits and vegetables every day

It's more important for healthy individuals to eat for continued overall health than to try to fashion a diet to ward off one particular disease. Willett said the bottom line is that almost everyone is at substantial risk for cardiovascular disease, and a diet that protects against cardiovascular disease is also good for cancer prevention. Lowering blood cholesterol reduces the risk of heart disease. Cholesterol in the diet comes only from foods from animal sources such as meat, dairy, eggs, and animal fats. Eating fewer animal products and eating more fiber—beans, vegetables, whole grains, and fruits are all good sources—helps lower blood cholesterol.

Fruits and Vegetables

The idea that foods may play a role in reducing the risk of cancer first emerged based on findings that linked fruit and vegetable consumption with lower cancer risk. In the majority of scientific studies on this subject, greater consumption of vegetables, fruits, or both has been associated with a lower risk of lung, esophageal, oral, stomach, and colon cancers. Evidence is less strong that eating fruits and vegetables prevents hormonally related types of cancers like breast and prostate.

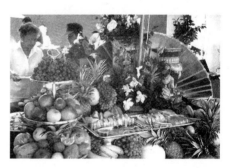

Eating five or more servings of vegetables and fruits each day is a healthful habit. Photo courtesy of Dr. Edwin P. Ewing, Jr., and the Centers for Disease Control and Prevention.

In general, the brightest-colored fruits and vegetables—green, red, yellow, and orange—tend to contain the most nutrients, including *antioxidants*. Antioxidants are nutrients in fruits and vegetables that appear to protect against the constant tissue damage that occurs during normal metabolism. Because such damage is associated with increased cancer risk, antioxidant nutrients are thought to protect against cancer. Antioxidants include *vitamin C*, *vitamin E*, *selenium*, *carotenoids* (relatives of vitamin A), and some other *phytochemicals* (chemicals from plants) that occur naturally in plant foods.

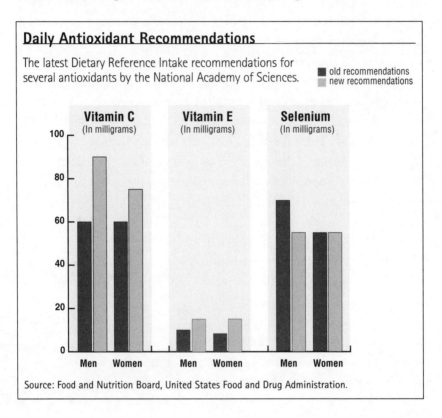

Daily Antioxidant Recommendations

The latest Dietary Reference Intake recommendations for several antioxidants by the National Academy of Sciences.

- old recommendations
- new recommendations

Source: Food and Nutrition Board, United States Food and Drug Administration.

Soy

Some studies suggest that consuming soy products (products made from soybeans, like tofu, soy milk, and soy powder) may reduce the risk of breast and prostate cancer, but more research is needed. Soy contains several phytochemicals, some of which appear to protect against hormone-dependent cancers in animal studies. High doses of soy supplements, on the other hand, could theoretically increase the risk of estrogen-responsive cancers, such as breast or endometrial cancer.

Phytochemicals at a Glance

Plants produce a wide variety of compounds called phytochemicals. These are compounds in fruits, vegetables, beans, grains, and other plants. The information below shows some of the phytochemicals that occur naturally in foods and may have cancer-fighting effects.

Researchers are trying to determine which of the thousands of phytochemicals are most effective for disease prevention. The best way to get a balance of phytochemicals is to eat a mostly plant-based diet, which includes at least five servings of a variety of fruits and vegetables each day.

Phytochemical	Source	Potential Benefits
Beta carotene	Carrots, squash, sweet potatoes, dark green leafy vegetables such as spinach, and many fruits	May be an effective cancer-preventing nutrient, although supplements have been found to increase the risk of lung cancer among smokers
Ascorbic acid (Vitamin C)	Citrus fruits, green leafy vegetables, potatoes, strawberries, bell peppers, and cantaloupe	Many studies have shown a connection between eating foods rich in vitamin C and a reduced risk of certain cancers
Lycopene	Tomatoes, apricots, guava, watermelon, papaya, and pink grapefruit	Diets rich in tomatoes, which contain lycopene, appear to protect cells from damage and may lower the risk of certain types of cancer, especially prostate, lung, and stomach cancer
Folic acid	Dark leafy green vegetables, citrus fruit, poultry, liver, and fortified grain-based cereals	Folic acid may reduce the risk of some cancers, including colon cancer
Vitamin E	Vegetable oils (especially safflower oil, sunflower oil, and cottonseed oil), green leafy vegetables, nuts, cereals, meats, egg yolks, wheat germ, and whole-wheat products	There is some evidence of the protective effects of vitamin E against prostate and colorectal cancer, but studies overall have been inconclusive
Ellagic acid	Raspberries, blackberries, cranberries, strawberries, pecans, pomegranates, and walnuts	Is believed to have anticancer effects; has been shown to slow the growth of tumors in animal studies
Sulphoraphane	Broccoli	Can encourage the body to produce protective enzymes that may prevent the cell damage that can lead to cancer

Fiber

People who eat a lot of fruits and vegetables reduce their risk of cancer. Researchers are not sure if it is the fiber that is responsible for this difference or other nutrients in the fruits and vegetables. Beans and whole-wheat products are also good sources of fiber.

Whole Grains

A whole grain is made up of three parts: the bran, endosperm, and germ. Processed, or refined, grains are made from only the endosperm. Because the bran and germ contain much of the vitamins, minerals, and all of the fiber found in grains, whole grains have more fiber and nutrients than refined grains. Whole grains not only provide the body with important nutrients, they can also help keep weight down. Refined carbohydrates, such as pastries, sweetened cereals, soft

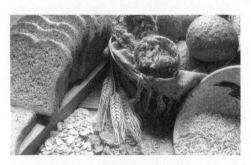

drinks, and sugars add calories but not many nutrients to your diet.

"It may be harder to control your weight on a high-carbohydrate, high-sugar diet," Willett says. "You absorb carbohydrates very quickly and you become hungry again." He notes that whole grains take longer to digest and keep you satisfied longer.

Whole grains provide important nutrients. Photo courtesy of the National Cancer Institute.

Meat and Fish

The major source of saturated fat and cholesterol in the American diet comes from foods derived from animal sources, especially meats like beef, pork, and lamb. Even though red meat is an excellent source of protein and certain vitamins and minerals, these nutrients can be obtained from other foods. In general, it's best to limit consumption of red meats and processed meats such as hot dogs, bacon, sausage, salami, and bologna. Instead, choose fish, poultry, or beans as an alternative. When you do eat red meat, select lean cuts and eat smaller portions.

Some evidence suggests that the way meat is cooked can affect its cancer-causing potential. Frying or charcoal-broiling meat at very high temperatures creates chemicals that cause cancer in animal experiments, but it's not clear whether they actually cause cancer in people. It may be wise for people to limit how often they grill meats and to avoid eating the charred parts. Instead, choose meats that have been baked, broiled, or poached.

Animal studies have found that the *omega-3 fatty acids* (nutrients involved in many body processes) found in fish may suppress cancer formation. There is limited evidence of a possible benefit in humans. It has not been proven that the possible benefits of fish consumption are reproducible through omega-3 or fish oil supplements.

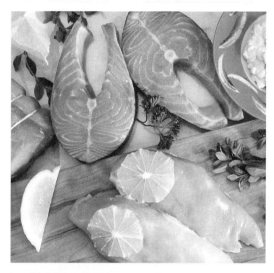

Lean beef, fish, and poultry are excellent sources of protein. However, it is wise to limit consumption of red meat and processed meats. Photo courtesy of the National Cancer Institute.

Fats

Many people who are on diets or who are conscious about maintaining their weight are worried about fat. Eating too much fat can hurt your health, but fat is a necessary nutrient. Among the many essential functions it serves, fat helps the body absorb certain vitamins, stores energy, helps maintain hair and skin, and protects vital organs.

High-fat diets have been associated with an increase in the risk of cancers of the colon, rectum, prostate, and endometrium. (The association between dietary fat and breast cancer risk is not as strong.) Whether these associations are due to the total amount of fat, type of fat, or the high number of calories in fatty food—or some other factor—has not yet been conclusively determined. The relationship of dietary fat to cancer risk is being actively studied.

The Skinny on Fat

According to the *Lahey Clinic Health Magazine*, *fatty acids* are chains of carbon atoms, with varying numbers of hydrogen atoms. *Saturated fats* are loaded, or saturated, with hydrogen atoms. This causes the molecule to be stiff and straight and allows the molecules to stack neatly and compactly, resulting in a solid. Animal fat is primarily saturated, as are certain tropical vegetable oils such as palm kernel and coconut oils.

	Saturated Fats	Monounsaturated Fats
Examples	Butter/shortening, egg yolks, chocolate, dairy products, meats and poultry with skin, palm and coconut oil	Olive, canola, and peanut oils; avocados; plant foods; some seafood
Effect	Raises blood cholesterol In combination with high-carbohydrate and high-calorie diets, may increase risk of cancer and heart disease	May lower blood cholesterol May lessen the risk of heart disease
What You Should Do	Cut back on foods from this list	Choose more of your fat-containing foods from this list

Although fat consumption is down to about 34 percent of calories in the average American diet compared to 40 percent a few years ago, Americans continue to eat far too many calories despite (or because of) the increased availability of fat-free and reduced-fat foods. "Low-fat" or "nonfat" just reflects the fat content of a food. It's also important to pay attention to the number of calories in a food.

All fats are not created equal. There are several kinds of fat in our diets, and many foods contain a combination of types of fats. Current evidence indicates that trans fats and saturated fats in combination with high-carbohydrate and high-calorie diets may increase the risk for cancer as well as for heart disease.

If two hydrogen atoms are missing, the fat is known as *mono-unsaturated*. It bends, won't stack, and becomes liquid. Olive, peanut, and canola oil are primarily monounsaturated.

Take away more hydrogen atoms, and the fat is *polyunsaturated*. These molecules bend in several places, making them more liquid. Most vegetable oils and fish oils are primarily polyunsaturated.

A food-industry process called hydrogenation adds hydrogen to an unsaturated fat, such as vegetable oil. The resulting *trans fat* has straight molecules that stack into a semi-solid, making it spreadable like margarine.

Polyunsaturated Fats	Trans Fats
Corn, soybean, sesame, and safflower oils; plant foods; some seafood	Partially hydrogenated vegetable oils, beef, pork, lamb, dairy products, many fast foods and baked goods, including most commercially produced white breads
May lower blood cholesterol May lessen the risk of heart disease	Raises blood cholesterol In combination with high-carbohydrate and high-calorie diets, may increase risk of cancer and heart disease
Choose more of your fat-containing foods from this list	Limit intake of foods from this list

Sugar

Sugar increases caloric intake without providing any of the nutrients that reduce cancer risk. By promoting obesity and elevating levels of insulin (hormones that regulate sugar levels in the blood), high sugar intake may increase cancer risk. White (refined) sugar, raw (unrefined) sugar, and honey have the same effects on body weight or insulin.

According to an article in the *Atlanta Journal-Constitution*, 19 November 2002, a review conducted by the food and nutrition panel of the National Academy of Sciences cited five studies showing higher incidence of colorectal cancer among heavy sugar users.

(The panel did note, however, that the risk is lower for those who get their sugar from fiber-loaded sources such as fruit.) Another study suggested that sugar-rich, fiber-poor foods are also associated with an increased risk of lung cancer.

Additionally, researchers are looking into the role of a particular insulin-like growth-factor system in the development of several types of cancer. (A *growth factor* is a naturally occurring protein that causes cells to grow and divide. Too much growth factor production by some cancer cells helps them grow quickly.)

Tea and Coffee

Some researchers have theorized that tea might protect against cancer because it contains antioxidants. In animal studies, some teas (including green tea) have been shown to reduce cancer risk, but tea has not been proven to reduce cancer risk in humans.

Caffeine may heighten some women's likelihood of developing of *fibrocystic breast lumps*—benign lumps in breast tissue that respond to female hormones. There is no evidence that caffeine increases the risk of breast cancer or other types of cancer. Some older, widely publicized studies suggested that coffee consumption might be a risk factor for pancreatic cancer, but most recent studies have not confirmed this theory.

Vegetarian Diets

Vegetarian diets include many health-promoting features. They tend to be low in saturated fat and high in fiber, vitamins, and phyto-chemicals. But a vegetarian diet isn't proven to have any special effects for the prevention of cancer.

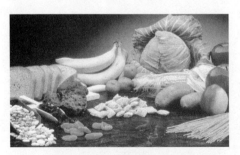

Fruits, vegetables, and grains are all important parts of a vegetarian diet. Photo courtesy of the National Cancer Institute.

Vegetarian diets differ (for example, some exclude dairy and/or eggs in addition to meat, fowl, and fish), although all avoid red meat. A vegetarian diet can be very healthy if it is carefully planned and provides adequate calories. But the greater the restriction of food groups in a particular diet, the more possibility there is of dietary deficiencies. Strict vegetarians should take supplements for vitamin B12, zinc, and iron, which may be missing from vegetarian diets.

Bioengineered Foods

Bioengineered foods are made by adding genes from other plants or other organisms to increase a plant's resistance to pests, to slow spoilage, or to improve transportability, flavor, nutrient composition, or other desired qualities. In theory, these added genes might create substances that could cause adverse reactions among sensitized or allergic individuals. There is currently no evidence, however, that the substances found in bioengineered foods now on the market are harmful or that the added genes would either increase or decrease cancer risk.

Food Additives

Many substances are added to foods to preserve them and to enhance color, flavor, and texture. Additives are usually present in very small quantities in food, and no convincing evidence has shown that any additive at these levels causes human cancers.

Dietary Supplements

The term *dietary supplement* includes vitamins, minerals, herbs, amino acids, and other products that, according to current regulations, are not considered to be "drugs." At this time, no evidence exists that supplements can reduce cancer risk.

Studies of antioxidant supplements have not shown a reduction in cancer risk. In fact, beta-carotene supplements have been associated with a higher risk of lung cancer in cigarette smokers.

Many healthful compounds exist in vegetables and fruits, and these compounds most likely add to these foods' beneficial effect. There are likely to be important, but as yet unidentified, components of whole food that are not included in supplements. To reduce cancer risk, it's best to consume vitamins, minerals, and antioxidants through food sources, rather than through supplements.

Think Before You Drink

Studies clearly show that cancer risk increases with the amount of alcohol consumed, whether it is hard liquor, wine, or beer. A person's choice of alcoholic beverage may be less important than how much that person drinks.

The ACS advises men to limit alcohol to two drinks a day; women are advised to have a maximum of one drink a day. A drink is defined as twelve ounces of regular beer, five ounces of wine, or one and a half ounces of 80-proof liquor.

Cancer risk substantially increases with even moderate drinking, defined as more than two drinks per day. Alcohol consumption increases the risk for cancers of the mouth, throat, esophagus, liver, and, for women, the breast. It may also be related to the risk of colorectal cancer.

Researchers don't know exactly why alcohol increases cancer risk. Some researchers believe that alcohol may bring about changes in hormones in the blood. It's also possible that alcohol and the substances produced in its breakdown might have a cancer-causing effect on tissues, for example, in the breast. According to a Mayo Clinic study, the cancer risk from drinking alcohol may be especially high for women who drink every day and whose mother, sisters, or daughters have breast cancer. Another possibility is that people who drink have lower levels of *folic acid*, a B vitamin that plays a key role in maintaining healthy DNA.

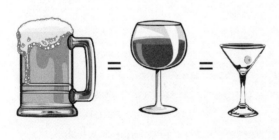

A bottle of beer, a glass of wine, a shot of liquor, and a mixed drink all have about the same amount of alcohol in them.

For some people, especially men over 50 and women over 60, the heart-protective benefits of *moderate* drinking may outweigh the risk of cancer. But there is no compelling reason for those who do not drink alcohol to start drinking. Discuss your risk factors for both heart disease and cancer with your health care team and make an informed decision about your own use of alcohol.

Keep Moving and Stay Trim

Regular physical activity can help protect against some cancers by burning off excess calories and preventing weight gain, by affecting hormone levels, and in other ways that are currently being studied.

Taking in too many calories and being physically inactive can cause a person to retain excess weight or become obese and can increase his or her risk for cancers at several sites, including the colon, esophagus, endometrium, breast (in postmenopausal women), kidney, pancreas, and gallbladder.

On the other hand, research has shown that people who exercise have a lower risk of colon and breast cancer. For example, a study by Dutch researchers found that active women had a 30 percent lower risk of breast cancer when compared to those who were inactive. Physical activity may also influence the risk for other cancers, but more research is needed to prove this definitively.

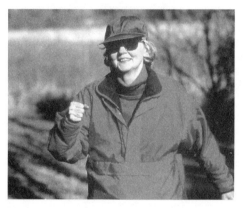

Regular physical activity can help protect against some types of cancer. Photo courtesy of the National Cancer Institute.

Take Stock of Your Body

Many factors influence weight, including genes (which play a direct role in determining height, body frame, and shape), activity level, age, and the amount and type of foods eaten. Because these factors vary from person to person, weight alone may not be a good indicator for risk of disease. People can use a number of different methods to determine if they are overweight or obese and therefore at increased risk for disease and disability.

Can Diet and Activity Reduce Your Risk of Cancer?

Type of Cancer	Convincing Evidence of Reducing Cancer Risk
Colorectal cancer	Physical activity Avoiding being overweight
Breast cancer	Physical activity Avoiding being overweight
Prostate cancer	
Lung cancer	
Stomach cancer	
Oral and esophageal cancer	Limiting alcohol intake
Bladder cancer	
Pancreatic cancer	
Endometrial cancer	Avoiding being overweight

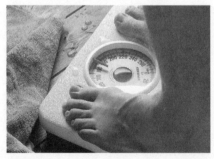

The body mass index is a ratio of weight to height. Photo courtesy of Bill Branson and the National Cancer Institute.

Body mass index (BMI) is probably the single best indicator of a person's amount of body fat. The BMI formula uses weight and height to determine levels of body fat for adults aged 20 and older.

Body mass index is really a ratio of weight to height. You can't change your height, but you can modify your weight (especially if your ratio is not

Probable Evidence of Reducing Cancer Risk	Possible Evidence of Reducing Cancer Risk
Eating lots of fruits and vegetables Limiting intake of red meats	Limiting alcohol intake
Limiting alcohol intake	Eating lots of fruits and vegetables
	Eating lots of fruits and vegetables
Limiting intake of red meats	
Eating lots of fruits and vegetables	
Eating lots of fruits and vegetables	
Avoiding being overweight Eating lots of fruits and vegetables	
	Eating lots of fruits and vegetables
	Eating lots of fruits and vegetables
Limiting intake of red meats	
	Limiting alcohol intake Avoiding being overweight
Physical activity	Eating lots of fruits and vegetables

within the healthy range of 18.5 to 25 kg/m2). Technically, BMI is your weight in kilograms divided by your height in meters squared. But it is much easier to determine BMI by using a chart, such as the one included here.

Keep in mind that people who are over the normal weight limits for their group but are very muscular are not necessarily overweight, because muscle weighs more than fat. Likewise, those at or below the weight standard for their height may have excessive body fat and little muscle. The BMI can be used as a general measure to help you maintain a healthy weight throughout life.

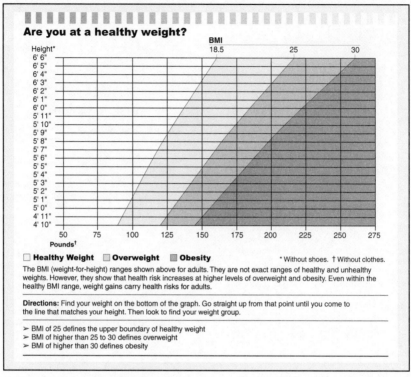

Are you at a healthy weight?

Table reprinted from *The Report of the Dietary Guidelines Advisory Committee on the Dietary Guidelines for Americans, 2000,* United States Department of Agriculture.

The Bottom Line

"People [with cancer] sometimes ask, 'Why me? What did I do?'" observes Eugenia Calle, Ph.D., director of analytical epidemiology for the ACS.

"There's not necessarily going to be a single answer for that question. In most cases, it's a complex series of cellular events that lead to cancer, and you can't single out one cause. We are wonderful beings, but there are many cells in the body and when they are dividing, sometimes they are going to make mistakes. All you can do is keep informed and adopt healthy habits. Hopefully, you'll live longer — but you'll definitely live better."

Conclusion

THE LONG HISTORY OF OUR STRUGGLE to understand cancer has led us in important new directions. We know many factors that affect our cancer risk, and we know which populations are most at risk for some types of cancer. Advancements in gene research allow us to understand important elements in cell growth and how malfunctions in them can lead to cancer. Environmental factors play a role as well. And we now know that lifestyle choices such as diet, exercise, and the use of alcohol or tobacco products contribute to a very large percentage of cancer cases.

By far the majority of cancers seem to be caused by complex inter-actions of genetics and environmental factors. Researchers are working to figure out exactly what causes a cell to develop into cancer.

"We're moving forward with lightning speed," says Robert Weinberg, Ph.D., a professor of biology at the Massachusetts Institute of Technology and a member of the Whitehead Institute for Biomedical Research in Cambridge, Massachusetts. "We've come a long way, but the many discoveries being made raise more and more questions."

According to Weinberg, these fundamental questions concerning the biology of what causes cancer include:

- How many different genes must be damaged before a cell will behave malignantly?

- How do different damaged genes collaborate with one another to create damaged cells?

- How do cells become invasive, or metastatic?

- Does cancer conform to a set of basic universal rules? Or does each cancer in every patient invent its own way of becoming malignant?

"These are not mysteries that are beyond solving with the techniques that we have today and the minds that we have working on the problem," Weinberg adds. "Within the next decade, most of these questions will be largely answered, but none of them will be completely answered."

Where Are We Now?

During the past few decades, scientists have made exciting discoveries with practical effects that have directly reduced cancer mortality rates.

Chemotherapy is a good example. Conventional cancer chemotherapy, first introduced in the 1950s, has made childhood leukemia curable in 90 percent of cases. But as noted, conventional cancer chemotherapy still kills healthy cells along with cancerous ones, causing side effects like nausea, vomiting, diarrhea, hair loss, and fatigue. This has been the story of almost all major medical advances: progress is made in fits and starts, and advances are gained only in the face of many obstacles.

Mindful of such mixed outcomes and the many lives at stake, scientists press ahead with two goals in mind. The first is to find a cure, to unmask the myriad causes of cancer so scientists can stop the disease before it starts. In the meantime, while they search for a cure, they focus on the second goal: to find better treatment options to improve the prognosis and quality of life for those who have already been diagnosed.

So where is cancer research headed? What discoveries may change our understanding of what causes cancer? What might aid our ability to detect, treat, and ultimately prevent cancer?

New Frontiers

Researchers continue to uncover promising links between causes, treatment, and prevention. Finding more effective cancer treatments gives us clues about how and why cancer forms, which in turn leads to better prevention and screening. We've already touched on some of the latest research into cancer and what causes it. Before we close, let's take a quick look at some of the most promising new directions in cancer research, as identified by Harmon Eyre, M.D., chief medical officer and executive vice president for research and cancer control at the American Cancer Society.

Chemoprevention

Chemoprevention is the use of natural or laboratory-made substances to reduce the risk of developing cancer. Researchers now know that there are compounds that can intervene in the transformation of a normal cell into a cancer cell, effectively stopping cancer before it starts. These range from compounds found in nature—such as those in broccoli, soy, and tea—as well as synthetic agents such as Nolvadex (generic name tamoxifen). Although scientists have some evidence that certain compounds may help prevent cancer in certain high-risk populations, they do not yet know if chemoprevention can help reduce the risk of cancer in the general population. The hope is that chemoprevention strategies can be tailored to prevent or stall the development of cancer in susceptible individuals long before invasive disease sets in.

Early Detection

The development of new and more accurate cancer screening methods will allow earlier detection of cancer, thereby enabling physicians to catch it before the disease progresses. For example, certain abnormal proteins that are involved in cancer seem to show up fairly consistently in the blood of people known to have cancer. Scientists are currently working to develop molecular tests to identify these *biomarkers* (substances that show up when particular processes are happening in the body) for cancer.

Chemotherapy

Chemotherapy uses medications that attack cells that divide quickly, whether they are cancerous or not. Using information gained from decades of studying the biology of cancer cells at the molecular level, researchers are learning how to focus a drug's attack on only cancer cells. This targeted approach is typified by Gleevec and drugs like it (see chapter 3), which leave normal cells largely unharmed, thus causing fewer side effects than traditional cancer therapies. New chemotherapy drugs, new combinations of drugs, and new delivery techniques hold significant promise for curing or controlling cancer and improving the quality of life for people already diagnosed.

Photodynamic Therapy

Photodynamic therapy (PDT) is a treatment that combines a light source and a *photosensitizing agent* (a drug that is activated by light) to destroy cancer cells. Clinical trials have shown that PDT can be as effective as surgery or radiation therapy in treating certain kinds of cancers and precancerous conditions, and has potentially fewer side effects. Another possible advantage is that therapy can be repeated several times at the same site if necessary.

Biologic Therapy

Biologic therapy is designed to stimulate or restore the body's ability to fight disease and infection. Think of it as a kind of immune-system boost.

Oncolytic viruses have oncolytic, or cancer-killing, properties — either naturally or because of laboratory manipulation. Designed to selectively infect cancer cells without harming healthy cells, the viruses replicate within the cancer cells, killing them. Far more remains to be understood about the potential and safety of this type of biologic therapy, which is being tested on several different cancers.

Immunotherapy is a type of biologic therapy that stimulates the natural defenses of your immune system to fight diseases, including cancer. Immunotherapy is sometimes used by itself, but it is most often used along with another type of therapy to add to the anti-cancer effects of the main therapy.

One approach uses *monoclonal antibodies*, which are made in the laboratory and injected into patients, to seek out and destroy cancer cells that contain excess amounts of certain proteins. A second type of immunotherapy that shows promise is the use of *cancer vaccines*. Vaccines for cancer work much like traditional vaccines against infectious diseases. Unlike vaccines for infections, however, most cancer vaccines are designed for treatment rather than prevention. Containing substances derived from cancer cells, they trigger the body's immune system to respond against cancer cells already in the body.

Researchers have made significant progress in this field in the past few years, and many are optimistic that more effective immunotherapies can be developed to provide cancer treatment that is targeted, effective, and largely free of side effects.

Gene Therapy

Gene therapy involves inserting a specific gene into mutated cells to restore a missing function or to give the cells a new function. Gene therapy can be used to fight cancer in many different ways:

Adding Genes

- Adding functional genes to cells that have abnormal or missing genes.

- Adding genes to cancer cells to make them more vulnerable to chemotherapy or radiation.

- Adding genes to tumor cells so the cancerous cells are more easily detected and destroyed by the body's immune system.

- Adding genes to immune system cells to make the immune system better able to detect cancer cells.

- Adding angiogenesis (the process of blood vessel formation) inhibitor genes to cancer cells to cut off tumors' blood supply, stopping them from growing or even shrinking them.

Stopping or Blocking Genes

- Stopping oncogenes or other genes essential to cancer from working (stopping these genes or the proteins they make may prevent cancer from growing or spreading).

- Blocking genes that allow cancer cells to become resistant to chemotherapy drugs.

- Stopping genes that contribute to angiogenesis.

Gene therapy shows so much promise for fighting cancer that most gene therapy clinical trials are now cancer related. Although gene therapy has had some success, it is currently available only through participation in a clinical trial. It will probably be several years before gene therapy is ready for use in the general public.

Daily Decisions

Cancer research is enormously promising, but it isn't the only answer to eliminating cancer as a major health problem, points out Robert Young, M.D., national volunteer president of the American Cancer Society and president of Fox Chase Cancer Center in Philadelphia. The role that individuals can play in the battle against cancer is also important.

If everyone understood the causes of cancer and adjusted their lifestyle to reduce their risks (including reducing tobacco use, weight gain, and sun exposure, and increasing physical activity), the cancer mortality rate could be slashed by 50 percent during the next decade, says Weinberg.

"As a cancer researcher I can tell you that by changing lifestyles, the effects on cancer mortality will be vastly greater than anything that I or my colleagues can think up," he says. "Preventing a disease is far more effective than treating a disease once it has appeared. At least for the next generation—and probably for the next century—prevention will be vastly more useful than advances in therapy. One cannot overstate the importance of changes in lifestyle."

Making Progress

According to Richard D. Klausner, M.D., director of the National Cancer Institute (NCI), the United States is making progress controlling cancer.

"In the last decade, for the first time since we have been keeping records of cancer statistics, the rates of both new cancers and deaths from cancer have fallen," Klausner says.

Although rates of some cancers, like melanoma skin cancer, continue to rise, the good news is that more people are getting screened for breast, cervical, and colorectal cancers, boosting their chances of early detection. In addition, more practitioners are adopting state-of-the-art cancer treatments, thus helping to lower mortality rates.

And as we've seen in this chapter, researchers continue to make progress too. "New" methods of cancer prevention, detection, and treatment have their roots in research that has been going on for decades, but it's adding up to a rapid breakthrough rate and tremendous potential for the coming years.

"Much of what we've learned is coming to fruition now," says Young. "This accumulation of understanding has revolutionized the way we deal with this disease and how we see ourselves conquering it eventually."

"We're on the right track," agrees oncologist and cancer researcher Brian J. Druker, M.D., the JELD-WEN chair of Leukemia Research at the Oregon Health and Science University Cancer Institute. "We have great hope and optimism for the future," he continues, "but we can't be complacent. We must seize the momentum now."

Resources

American Cancer Society

The American Cancer Society (ACS) is the nationwide community-based volunteer health organization dedicated to eliminating cancer as a major health problem by preventing cancer, saving lives and diminishing suffering from cancer, through research, education, advocacy, and service. For more information about cancer, educational materials, patient programs, and services within your community, contact us:

Toll-free: 800-ACS-2345 (800-227-2345)

Web site: *http://www.cancer.org*

About the Resources

Listings in this section represent organizations that operate on a national level and provide some type of service or resource to consumers related to cancer, cancer research, or public health. This list is designed to offer a starting point for seeking information, support, and needed resources. Most of the organizations listed here can be contacted via phone, fax, or e-mail, and some through a Web site. Many of the Web sites provide much of the same information that is available by postal mail. Some organizations are solely Web-based and will require Internet access. Keep in mind that new Web sites appear daily while old ones expand, move, or disappear entirely. Some of the Web sites or content outlined below may change. Often, a simple Internet search will point to the new Web site for a given organization. The American Cancer Society Web site provides links to outside sources of cancer information as well (*http://www.cancer.org*; click on Cancer Resource Center).

There is a vast amount of information on the Internet. This information can be very valuable to the general public in making decisions about their health. However, since any group of individual can publish on the Internet, it is important to consider the credentials and reputation of the organization providing information. Internet information should not be a substitute for medical advice.

The American Cancer Society does not necessarily endorse the agencies, organizations, corporations, and publications represented in this resource guide. This guide is provided for assistance in obtaining information only.

Organizations Providing Health and Cancer Information

Agency for Healthcare Research and Quality (AHRQ)
Office of Health Care Information, Executive Office Center
2101 East Jefferson Street, Suite 501
Rockville, MD 20852
Phone: 301-594-1360
Web site: *http://www.ahrq.gov*
The AHRQ, an office within the U.S. Department of Health and Human Services (see page 193), provides consumers with science-based, easily understandable information that will help them make informed decisions about their own health care. They offer a number of clinical practice guidelines on common health problems in consumer versions for the public.

American College of Surgeons (ACoS) Commission on Cancer
633 North Saint Clair Street
Chicago, IL 60611-3211
Phone: 312-202-5000; 312-202-5085 Cancer Programs
Fax: 312-202-5009 or 5011
Web site: *http://www.facs.org*
The ACoS' Commission on Cancer accredits cancer programs of health care organizations in the United States. This voluntary approval program includes a site visit to evaluate the program's compliance with specific standards in ten major areas—from prevention to end-of-life care.

National Cancer Data Base (NCDB)
Web site: *http://www.facs.org/dept/cancer/ncdb*
The NCDB is a nationwide oncology outcomes database for close to 1,500 health care facilities with approved cancer programs in 50 states. It is estimated that close to 80 percent of newly diagnosed cases of cancer are submitted annually to the NCDB, which is jointly supported by the ACS and the ACoS' Commission on Cancer.

American Institute for Cancer Research (AICR)
1759 R Street NW
Washington, DC 20009
Toll-Free: 800-843-8114
Phone: 202-328-7744
Fax: 202-328-7226
Web site: *http://www.aicr.org*
The AICR supports research into the role of diet and nutrition in the prevention and treatment of cancer. It also offers a wide range of cancer prevention education programs and publications for health professionals and the public.

Cancer Research Institute (CRI)
681 Fifth Avenue
New York, NY 10022
Toll-Free: 800-99-CANCER (800-992-2623)
Phone: 212-688-7515
Fax: 212-688-7515
Web site: *http://www.cancerresearch.org*
CRI supports research aimed at developing new immunologic methods of diagnosing, treating, and preventing cancer. CRI can answer questions about cancer immunology and provide assistance in locating clinical trials studying immunotherapy.

Centers for Disease Control and Prevention (CDC)
Public Inquiries/MASO
MS F07
1600 Clifton Road NE
Atlanta, GA 30333
Phone: 404-639-3534
Toll-free: 800-311-3435
Web site: *http://www.cdc.gov*
The CDC is an agency of the U.S. Department of Health and Human Services (HHS) (see page 193). Their mission is to promote health and quality of life by preventing and controlling disease, injury, and disability. Their Web site contains a searchable map of the 12 centers, offices, and institutes; information about health topics; downloadable publications; and links to related sources. Listed below are some agencies of interest.

National Center for Chronic Disease Prevention and Health Promotion (NCCDPHP)
4770 Buford Highway NE
MS K64
Atlanta, GA 30341
Toll-free: 888-842-6355
Phone: 770-488-5820
Web site: *http://www.cdc.gov/nccdphp*
The NCCDPHP prevents premature death and disability from chronic diseases and promotes healthy personal behaviors. The NCCDPHP houses eight divisions, some of which are listed below.

Division of Cancer Prevention and Control (DCPC)
Web site: *http://www.cdc.gov/cancer*
The DCPC conducts, supports, and promotes efforts to prevent cancer and to increase early detection of cancer. DCPC works with partners in the government, private, and nonprofit sectors to develop, implement, and promote effective cancer prevention and control practices nationwide.

National Program of Cancer Registries (NPCR)
Web site: *http://www.cdc.gov/cancer/npcr*
Cancer registry data collected through the NPCR are used to identify and monitor trends in cancer incidence and mortality; guide planning and evaluation of cancer control programs; help allocate health resources; contribute to clinical, epidemiologic, and health services research; and respond to concerns from citizens over the presence of cancer in their communities.

Division of Nutrition and Physical Activity (DNPA)
Web site: *http://www.cdc.gov/nccdphp/dnpa*
The DNPA provides science-based activities for children and adults that address the role of nutrition and physical activity in health promotion and the prevention and control of chronic diseases.

Office on Smoking and Health (OSH)
4770 Buford Highway NE
MS K50
Atlanta, GA 30341-3724
Toll-free: 800-232-1311 (800-232-1311) for prepared voice/fax information only
Phone: 770-488-5705
Web site: *http://www.cdc.gov/tobacco*
The OSH is responsible for leading and coordinating strategic efforts aimed at preventing tobacco use among youth, promoting tobacco cessation, and protecting nonsmokers from environmental tobacco smoke. The Web site offers public education and information on smoking and how to stop.

National Center for Environmental Health (NCEH)
4770 Buford Highway NE
Mail Stop F29
Atlanta, GA 30341-3724
Toll-free phone: 888-232-6789 for the NCEH Health Line
Web site: *http://www.cdc.gov/nceh*
The NCEH provides national leadership in preventing and controlling disease and death resulting from the interactions between people and their environment. The toll-free telephone number can be used for information and faxes on child-hood lead poisoning, cruise ship inspection, cholesterol measurements, and list of publications.

Office of Genomics and Disease Prevention
4770 Buford Highway NE
MS K28
Atlanta, GA 30341-3724
Phone: 770-488-3235
Fax: 770-488-3236
The Office of Genomics and Disease Prevention's goals are to promote leadership in genetic policy development, develop science for public health action, communicate and distribute information, and train and educate the public health workforce.

National Center for Health Statistics (NCHS)
6525 Belcrest Road
Hyattsville, MD 20782-2003
Phone: 301-458-4636
Web site: *http://www.cdc.gov/nchs*
The NCHS provides statistical information that will guide actions and policies to improve the health of the American people. The NCHS is the U.S. government's principal vital and health statistics agency. It provides a wide variety of data in order to monitor the nation's health.

National Institute for Occupational Safety and Health (NIOSH)
Hubert H. Humphrey Building
200 Independence Avenue SW
Room 715H
Washington, DC 20201
Toll-free: 800-35-NIOSH (800-356-4674)
Toll-free fax-on-demand: 888-232-3299
Web site: *http://www.cdc.gov/niosh*
The NIOSH ensures the safety and health for all people in the workplace through research and prevention. The NIOSH investigates potentially hazardous working conditions as requested by employers or employees. NIOSH information specialists and the NIOSH Web site provide information on many work safety topics, including lung diseases, cancer, asbestos and other chemical hazards, indoor air quality, electromagnetic fields, and personal protective equipment.

Environmental Protection Agency (EPA)
Ariel Rios Building
1200 Pennsylvania Avenue NW
Washington, DC 20460
Phone: 202-260-2090
Web site: *http://www.epa.gov*
The EPA implements the federal laws designed to promote public health by protecting our nation's air, water, and soil from harmful pollution. The Web site offers environmental news, community concerns, information about laws and other regulations, and links to other sources of information.

Office of Pesticide Programs (OPP)
Web site: *http://www.epa.gov/pesticides*
The mission of the OPP is to protect public health and the environment from the risks posed by pesticides and to promote safer means of pest control. The Web site provides consumer alerts, information about pesticides and their use and disposal, a kid's section, industry-related topics, and other information.

Office of Water (OW)
Safe Drinking Water Hotline: 800-426-4791
Web site: *http://www.epa.gov/water*
The OW is responsible for the EPA's water quality activities, including development of national programs, technical policies, and regulations relating to drinking water, water quality, ground water, pollution source standards, and the protection of wetlands, marine, and estuarine areas.

Food and Agriculture Organization of the United Nations (FAO)
Viale delle Terme di Caracalla, 00100
Rome, Italy
Phone: +39 06 5705 1
Fax: +39 06 5705 3152
Telex: 625852/610181 FAO I /
Web site: *http://www.fao.org*
The FAO of the United Nations was founded in 1945 with a mandate to raise levels of nutrition and standards of living, to improve agricultural productivity, and to better the condition of rural populations. Today, FAO is one of the largest specialized agencies in the United Nations system and the lead agency for agriculture, forestry, fisheries, and rural development.

Food and Drug Administration (FDA)
5600 Fishers Lane
Rockville, MD 20857-0001
Phone: 888-INFO-FDA (888-463-6332)
Fax: 301-443-9767
Web site: *http://www.fda.gov*
The FDA is an agency within the U.S. Department of Health and Human Services (see page 193) and consists of eight centers/offices, two of which are listed below. The FDA is a public health agency charged with protecting Americans by enforcing the Federal Food, Drug, and Cosmetic Act and other laws, promoting health by helping

safe and effective products reach the market in a timely way, and monitoring products for continued safety after they are in use. The FDA regulates food, cosmetics, medicines, biologics, medical devices, and radiation-emitting consumer products, as well as feed and drugs for pets and farm animals. The Web site has extensive information about all the products the FDA regulates.

Center for Biologics Evaluation and Research (CBER)
Food and Drug Administration
1401 Rockville Pike, Suite 200N
Rockville, MD 20852-1448
Toll-free: 800-835-4709
Phone: 301-827-1800
Fax: 301-827-3844
The CBER protects and enhances the public health through the regulation of biological and related products including blood, vaccines, tissue (for transplantation), cellular and gene therapy, allergenics and antitoxins, and biological therapeutics.

Center for Devices and Radiological Health (CDRH)
Food and Drug Administration
1350 Piccard Drive, HFZ-210
Rockville, MD 20850
Toll-free: 888-463-6332
Phone: 301-827-3990
Web site: *http://www.fda.gov/cdrh*
The CDRH provides information about the development, safety and effectiveness, and regulation of medical devices and electronic products that produce radiation. The center also monitors devices throughout the product life cycle, and it assures that radiation-emitting products, such as microwave ovens, TV sets, cell phones, and laser products, meet radiation safety standards.

Institute for Advanced Studies in Aging and Geriatric Medicine (IASIA)
1700 Wisconsin Avenue NW
First floor
Washington, DC 20007
Phone: 202-333-8845
Fax: 202-333-8898
Web site: *http://www.iasia.org*
The IASIA is a nonprofit biomedical research and educational organization that accelerates the pace of scientific discovery in human aging by both conducting clinical research and facilitating education by uniting researchers, educators, and clinicians.

Intercultural Cancer Council (ICC)
6655 Travis, Suite 322
Houston, TX 77030-1312
Phone: 713-798-4517
Fax: 713-798-6222
Web site: *http://iccnetwork.org*
The ICC promotes policies, programs, partnerships, and research to eliminate the unequal burden of cancer among racial and ethnic minorities and medically underserved populations in the United States and its associated territories.

International Epidemiology Institute (IEI)

1455 Research Boulevard, Suite 550

Rockville, MD 20850

Phone: 301-517-4060

Fax: 301-517-4063

Web site: *http://www.iei.ws*

The IEI is a biomedical research organization that offers its international experience in a range of epidemiologic services from the design and execution of investigations to the evaluation and presentation of study results to public and private sectors, universities, and other institutions, in order to understand the etiology and means of prevention of human illness.

National Academy of Sciences (NAS)

500 Fifth Street NW

Washington, DC 20001

Web site: *http://www.nationalacademies.org/nas*

The NAS is a private, nonprofit, self-perpetuating society of distinguished scholars engaged in scientific and engineering research, dedicated to the furtherance of science and technology and to their use for the general welfare.

National Cancer Institute (NCI)

NCI Public Inquiries Office

Building 31, Room 10A31

31 Center Drive, MSC 2580

Bethesda, MD 20892-2580

Toll-Free: 800-4-CANCER (800-422-6237)

Web site: *http://www.cancer.gov*

This government agency, as part of the National Institutes of Health (NIH) (see page 187) provides information on cancer research, diagnosis, and treatment through several services (see list below). People with cancer, caregivers, and health care professionals may call the NCI's toll-free telephone service for cancer-related information. *Spanish-speaking staff and Spanish materials are available.*

CancerFax

Toll-Free Fax: 800-624-2511

Fax: 301-402-5874

CancerFax includes information about cancer treatment, screening, prevention, and supportive care. To obtain a contents list, dial the fax number from a fax machine hand set and follow the recorded instructions.

Cancer Genome Anatomy Project (CGAP)

Web site: *http://cgap.nci.nih.gov*

The goal of the NCI's CGAP is to determine the gene expression profiles of normal, precancerous, and cancer cells, leading eventually to improved detection, diagnosis, and treatment for the patient. By collaborating with scientists world-wide, CGAP seeks to increase its scientific expertise and expand its databases for the benefit of all cancer researchers.

Cancer Information Service (CIS)

Toll-Free: 800-4-CANCER (800-422-6237)
Toll-Free (TTY): 800-332-8615
Web site: *http://cis.nci.nih.gov*
The CIS provides information to consumers and health care professionals. The Web site contains a wealth of information including pamphlets and brochures on cancer diagnosis, treatment, research, and prevention. *Spanish-speaking staff is available.*

CancerNet

Web site: *http://cancernet.gov*
Web site (Spanish version): *http://cancernet.gov/sp_menu.htm*
Web site (online ordering): *http://publications.nci.nih.gov*
CancerNet is a comprehensive Web site that contains information on diagnosis, treatment, support, resources, literature, clinical trials, prevention and risk factors, and testing. Up to twenty publications can be ordered online. The publications list is searchable. *Some publications are available in Spanish.*

Division of Cancer Epidemiology and Genetics (DCEG)

6130 Executive Boulevard
EPS Room 8070
Bethesda, MD 20892-7335
Phone: 301-496-1611
Fax: 301-402-3256
Web site: *http://dceg.cancer.gov*
The DCEG of the NCI serves as a national resource for population-based studies in cancer etiology and to identify environmental and genetic determinants of cancer. Research areas of special interest include genetic predisposition, lifestyle factors, environmental contaminants, occupational exposures, medications, radiation, and infectious agents, as well as statistics and methods development.

The Epidemiology and Biostatistics Program (EBP)

6120 Executive Boulevard
EPS Room 8094
Bethesda, Maryland 20892-7335
Phone: 301-496-3004
Fax: 301-402-8229
Web site: *http://dceg.cancer.gov/ebp/index.html*
The NCI's Epidemiology and Biostatistics Program (EBP) conducts independent and collaborative epidemiologic and biostatistical investigations to identify the distribution, characteristics, and causes of cancer in human populations. The Web site includes information about the EBP's areas of research, links to programs, and information about EBP studies.

The Long Island Breast Cancer Study Project (LIBCSP)
Division of Cancer Control and Population Sciences
National Cancer Institute
6130 Executive Boulevard
Executive Plaza North
Rockville, Maryland 20852
Phone: 301-594-6776
Fax: 301-594-6787
Web site: *http://epi.grants.cancer.gov/LIBCSP*
The Long Island Breast Cancer Study Project (LIBCSP) is a multistudy effort to
investigate whether environmental factors are responsible for breast cancer in Suffolk,
Nassau, and Schoharie counties, New York, and in Tolland County, Connecticut.
The investigation began in 1993 and is funded and coordinated by the NCI in collab-
oration with the National Institute of Environmental Health Sciences (NIEHS). The
LIBCSP Web site includes an overview of the study, statistics, and findings.

Office of Cancer Complementary and Alternative Medicine (OCCAM)
National Cancer Institute, NIH
6116 Executive Plaza North
Suite 600, MSC 8339
Bethesda, MD 20852
Toll-free: 888-NIH-NCAM (888-644-6226) for the National Center for
Complementary and Alternative Medicine (NCCAM) Clearinghouse
Web site: *http://www3.cancer.gov/occam*
The OCCAM coordinates and enhances the activities of the NCI in the arena of
complementary and alternative medicine. The goal of the OCCAM is to increase
the amount of high-quality cancer research and information about the use of
complementary and alternative modalities.

Surveillance, Epidemiology and End Results (SEER) Program
Cancer Statistics Branch
Surveillance Research Program
Division of Cancer Control and Population Sciences
National Cancer Institute
Suite 504, MSC 8316
6116 Executive Boulevard
Bethesda, MD 20892-8316
Phone: 301-496-8510
Fax: 301-496-9949
Email: cancer.gov_staff@mail.nih.gov
Web site: *http://www.seer.cancer.gov/*
The SEER Program is part of the NCI. Their Web site includes information
about cancer statistics and data collection tools.

National Center for Tobacco-Free Kids
1400 Eye Street, Suite 1200
Washington, DC 20005
Phone: 202-296-5469
Fax: 202-296-5427

E-mail: info@tobaccofreekids.org
Web site: *http://www.tobaccofreekids.org*
The National Center for Tobacco-Free Kids, also known as the Campaign for Tobacco-Free Kids, is an independent, nonpartisan, inclusive organization that works to prevent tobacco use by children and youth. The Web site has information about federal, state, and international initiatives, tobacco news, research, and how children can get involved in prevention tobacco use among their peers. The center works in partnership with the American Cancer Society, American Heart Association, American Medical Association, American Academy of Pediatrics, and 100 other health, civic, corporate, youth, and religious organizations.

National Consumers League
1701 K Street NW, Suite 1201
Washington, DC 20006
Phone: 202-835-3323
Fax: 202-835-0747
Web site: *http://www.nclnet.org*
Experts in law, business, and labor provide consumer protection and advocacy. The National Consumers League publishes education brochures about general health issues, including cancer-screening tests.

National Council Against Health Fraud
119 Foster Street
Peabody, MA 01960
Phone: 978-532-9383
Web site: *http://www.ncahf.org*
This private, nonprofit voluntary health agency focuses on health misinformation, fraud, and quackery, and provides information on unusual methods of cancer management. It can refer people to lawyers and help those who have had negative experiences to share their story.

National Institutes of Health (NIH)
9000 Rockville Pike
Bethesda, MD 20892
Mailing address: NIH
Building 1
1 Center Drive
Bethesda, Maryland 20892
Toll-free: 800-4-CANCER (800-422-6237); (TYY) 800-332-8615
Phone: 301-496-4000
Web site: *http://www.nih.gov*
The NIH is one of the world's foremost medical research centers, and the federal focal point for medical research in the United States. The NIH, comprised of 27 separate Institutes and Centers, is one of the eight health agencies of the Public Health Service, which, in turn, is part of the U.S. Department of Health and Human Services (HHS) (see page 193). The goal of NIH research is to acquire new knowledge to help prevent, detect, diagnose, and treat disease and disability, from the rarest genetic disorder to the common cold. The NIH mission is to uncover new knowledge that will lead to better health for everyone.

National Center on Minority Health and Health Disparities (NCMHHD)
6707 Democracy Boulevard
Suite 800, MSC-5465
Bethesda, MD 20892-5465
Phone: 301-402-1366; (TTY) 301 451-9532
FAX: 301-480-4049
The mission of the NCMHD is to promote minority health and to lead, coordinate, support, and assess the NIH effort to reduce and ultimately eliminate health disparities. The NCMHD conducts and supports basic, clinical, social, and behavioral research, promotes research infrastructure and training, fosters emerging programs, disseminates information, and reaches out to minority and other health disparity communities.

National Center for Complementary and Alternative Medicine (NCCAM)
NCCAM Clearinghouse
P.O. Box 8218
Silver Spring, MD 20907-8218
Toll-free: 888-644-6226; (TYY) 866-464-3615
Phone: 301-231-7537, ext. 5 (for calling from outside the U.S.)
Fax: 301-495-4957
Web site: *http://nccam.nih.gov*
This center provides research-based information on complementary and alternative methods being promoted to treat different diseases.

National Library of Medicine (NLM)
8600 Rockville Pike
Bethesda, MD 20894
Toll-free: 888-FIND-NLM (888-346-3656) for the Reference and Customer Service Telephone Desk
Phone: 301-594-5983
Fax: 301-402-1384
Web site: *http://www.nlm.nih.gov*
The NLM collects, organizes, and makes available biomedical science information to investigators, educators, and practitioners and carries out programs designed to strengthen medical library services in the United States. Its electronic databases are used extensively throughout the world by both health professionals and the public. *Materials are available in languages other than English.*

Internet Grateful Med
Web site: *http://igm.nlm.nih.gov*
This Internet-based service provides access to millions of literature references and abstracts in MEDLINE and other databases, with links to online journals. The site is searchable by keywords.

MEDLINEplus
Web site: *http://www.nlm.nih.gov/medlineplus/medlineplus*
MEDLINEplus is a database for consumer health information including dictionaries; articles and journals from other organizations; textbooks, newsletters, and health news for online reading; and links to organizations that provide consumer information and clearinghouses that send health literature.

NLM Gateway
Web site: *http://gateway.nlm.nih.gov/gw/Cmd*
The NLM Gateway offers links to searchable databases and allows users to search simultaneously in multiple retrieval systems.

PubMed
Web site: *http://www.ncbi.nlm.nih.gov/PubMed*
This database provides access to millions of literature references and abstracts in MEDLINE and other databases, with links to online journals. The site is searchable by keyword.

National Human Genome Research Institute (NHGRI)
Communications and Public Liaison Branch
Building 31, Room 4B09
31 Center Drive, MSC 2152
9000 Rockville Pike
Bethesda, MD 20892-2152
Phone: 301-402-0911
Fax: 301-402-2218
Web site: *http://www.genome.gov*
NHGRI supports the NIH component of the Human Genome Project, a worldwide research effort designed to analyze the structure and location of human DNA and genes. The NHGRI supports genetic and genomic research, investigation into the ethical, legal, and social implications surrounding genetics research, and educational outreach activities.

The Ethical, Legal, and Social Implications (ELSI) Program
National Human Genome Research Institute, NIH
Building 31, Room B2B07
31 Center Drive, MSC 2033
Bethesda, MD 20892-2033
Phone: 301-402-4997
Fax: 301-402-1950
Web site: *http://www.genome.gov/page.cfm?pageID=10001618*
The NHGRI's ELSI Program was established in 1990 as an integral part of the United States Human Genome Project (HGP (see page 194) to foster basic and applied research, and support education and outreach. The ELSI program funds and manages studies related to the ethical, legal, and social implications of genetic and genomic research, and supports workshops, research consortia, and policy conferences related to these topics.

National Institute on Aging (NIA)
Building 31, Room 5C27
31 Center Drive, MSC 2292
Bethesda, MD 20892-2292
Toll-free: 800-222-2225 for the Information Center
Phone: 301-496-1752
Web site: *http://www.nia.nih.gov*
The NIA leads a broad scientific effort to understand the nature of aging and to extend the healthy, active years of life. The NIA's mission is to improve the health and well-being of older Americans through research and public information.

National Institute of Environmental Health Sciences (NIEHS)
111 Alexander Drive
P.O. Box 12233
Research Triangle Park, NC 27709
Phone: 919-541-3345
Fax: 919-541-4395
Web site: *http://www.niehs.nih.gov/*
The mission of NIEHS is to reduce the burden of human illness and dysfunction from environmental causes by understanding each of these elements and how they interrelate. Their Web site includes information about environmental health news, programs run by the NIEHS, and an online library.

National Toxicology Program (NTP)
Web site: *http://ntp-server.niehs.nih.gov*
The NTP coordinates toxicology research and testing activities to provide information about potentially toxic chemicals to regulatory and research agencies and the public, and to strengthen the science base in toxicology. The NTP has become the world's leader in designing, conducting, and interpreting animal assays for toxicity/carcinogenicity and reproduction/development. The NTP's *Report on Carcinogens* identifies substances and mixtures or exposure circumstances that are "known" or are "reasonably anticipated" to cause cancer, and to which a significant number of Americans are exposed. The *Report on Carcinogens* is published every two years and is available on the NTP Web site.

Office of the Surgeon General
5600 Fishers Lane, Room 18-66
Rockville, MD 20857
Toll-free: 800-789-2547 for information, reports, and fact sheets
Web site: *http://www.surgeongeneral.gov*
The Office of the Surgeon General is part of the Office of Public Health and Science. It is also a part of the larger U.S. Department of Health and Human Services (see page 193). Reports of the Surgeon General and other publications are available via the Web site.

Secretary's Advisory Committee on Genetic Testing (SACGT)
Office of Biotechnology Activities, Office of Science Policy
National Institutes of Health
6705 Rockledge Drive

Suite 750, MSC 7985
Bethesda, MD 20892-7985 (All non-USPS mail should use zip code 20817)
Phone: 301-496-9838
Fax: 301-496-9839
Web site: *http://www4.od.nih.gov/oba/sacgt.htm*
The SACGT advises the government about all aspects of the development and
use of genetic tests, including the complex medical, ethical, legal, and social
issues raised by genetic testing. The SACGT is part of the Department of Health
and Human Services but is managed by the director of the NIH.

Women's Health Initiative (WHI)
Women's Health Initiative Program Office
1 Rockledge Centre
Suite 300, MS 7966
6705 Rockledge Drive
Bethesda, MD 20892-7966 (U.S. Postal Service)
Bethesda, MD 20817-7966 (Express Mail Service)
Phone: 301-402-2900
Fax: 301- 480-5158
Web site: *http://www.nhlbi.nih.gov/whi/index.html*
The Women's Health Initiative (WHI), the largest clinical trial ever undertaken in
the United States, addresses the most common causes of death, disability, and
impaired quality of life in postmenopausal women. It is expected that the WHI
will provide many answers concerning possible benefits and risks associated with
use of hormone replacement therapy, dietary supplements, and other interventions
in preventing cardiovascular disease, breast and colorectal cancer, and osteoporosis
in postmenopausal women.

National Safety Council (NSC)
1121 Spring Lake Drive
Itasca, IL 60143-3201
Toll-free: 800-621-7619
Phone: 630-285-1121
Fax: 630-285-1315
Web site: *http://www.nsc.org*
The NSC is a membership organization dedicated to protecting life and promoting
health. The Fact Sheet Library, available on the NSC Web site, provides over 80
handy resource guides offering statistics, tips, and suggestions for improving safety.

Radon Hotline
Toll-free: 800-557-2366 to speak to an information specialist
Toll-free: 800-767-7236 to request a brochure about radon
Web site: *http://www.nsc.org/ehc/radon.htm*
The National Safety Council in conjunction with the Environmental Health Center
has established a Radon Hotline to answer questions and provide materials about
radon, its health effects, and radon testing.

National Weather Service (NWS)
National Oceanic and Atmospheric Administration (NOAA)
1325 East-West Highway
Silver Spring, MD 20910
Web site: *http://www.nws.noaa.gov*
The NWS provides weather, hydrologic, and climate forecasts and warnings for the
United States, its territories, adjacent waters, and ocean areas for the protection of life
and property and the enhancement of the national economy. NWS data and products
include current weather and UV Index information, climate archives, statistical tables,
and links to other sites.

National Women's Health Information Center
The Office on Women's Health
U.S. Department of Health and Human Services
8550 Arlington Boulevard, Suite 300
Fairfax, VA 22031
Toll-Free: 800-994-WOMAN (800-994-9662); (TDD): 888-220-5546
Web site: *http://www.4woman.gov*
Web site (Spanish version): *http://www.4woman.gov/Spanish/index.htm*
This Web site has a searchable database of information on various women's health
issues, including breast cancer. Documents accessible through this site include infor-
mation from the NCI, the CDC, and several other government agencies. The site
contains a section for special groups, which separates breast cancer and other health
information by specific minority group. It also contains links to online medical dictionaries and journals.

Occupational Safety & Health Administration (OSHA)
U.S. Department of Labor
200 Constitution Avenue NW
Washington, DC 20210
Toll-free: 800-321-OSHA (800-321-6742)
Phone: 202-693-1999 (Public Affairs Office)
Web site: *http://www.osha.gov*
OSHA is responsible for creating and enforcing workplace safety and health regula-
tions to prevent work-related injuries, illnesses, and deaths. The OSHA Web site
includes: lists of known and suspected carcinogens, hazardous information bulletins,
and information on reproductive hazards.

Smoke-Free Kids, Inc.
P.O. Box 13886
Charleston, SC 29422
Phone: 843-588-0016
Fax: 843-588-0075
Web site: *http://www.jeffreywigand.com*
Smoke-Free Kids is the nonprofit foundation formed by Dr. Jeffrey Wigand, the
former chief scientist at Brown & Williamson Tobacco Corporation who went
public with what he knew about the tobacco industry.

Skin Cancer Foundation
245 Fifth Avenue, Suite 1403
New York, NY 10016
Toll-Free: 800-SKIN-490 (800-754-6490)
Fax: 212-725-5751
Web site: *http://www.skincancer.org*
The Skin Cancer Foundation conducts educational programs for the public and medical communities; supports medical training, cancer screening, and prevention programs; provides information about safe sun exposure for children and adults; and publishes a journal.

United States Census Bureau
4700 Silver Hill Road
Suitland, MD 20746
Mailing address: U.S. Census Bureau
Washington DC 20233
Phone: 301-763-INFO (4636) for the Call Center
Web site: *http://www.census.gov*
The Census Bureau's mission is to be the preeminent collector and provider of timely, relevant, and quality data about the people and economy of the United States.

United States Department of Health and Human Services (HHS)
200 Independence Avenue SW
Washington, DC 20201
Toll Free: 877-696-6775
Phone: 202-619-0257
Web site: *http://www.hhs.gov*
The Department of Health and Human Services (HHS) is the U.S. government's principal agency for protecting the health of all Americans and providing essential human services, especially for those who are least able to help themselves. One of the largest federal agencies, the HHS' responsibilities include public health (CDC, NIH, FDA, and others included), biomedical research, Medicare and Medicaid, welfare, social services, and more.

United States Department of Energy (DOE)
Office of Environment, Safety and Health (ES&H)
1000 Independence Avenue SW
Washington, DC 20585
Toll-free: 800-DIAL-DOE; 800-473-4375 for the ES&H Helpline
Fax: 202-586-4403
Web site: *http://portal.eh.doe.gov/communities/community.asp*
The ES&H is the DOE's advocate for excellence in programs to protect the environment, as well as the health and safety of workers at DOE facilities and the public.

United States Human Genome Project (HGP)
United States Department of Energy Human Genome Program
National Institutes of Health Human Genome Research Institute
Web site: *http://www.ornl.gov/hgmis*
The U.S. Human Genome Project (HGP), composed of the DOE and NIH Human
Genome Programs, is the national coordinated effort to characterize all human genet-
ic material by determining the complete sequence of the DNA in the human genome.
The HGP's ultimate goal is to discover all the more than 30,000 human genes and
render them accessible for further biological study. See also the National Human
Genome Research Institute (NHGRI), part of the NIH, and the Ethical, Legal, and
Social Implications (ELSI) Program.

World Health Organization (WHO)
WHO Headquarters
Avenue Appia 20
1211 Geneva 27
Switzerland
Phone: (+ 41 22) 791 21 11
Fax: (+ 41 22) 791 3111
United States Headquarters:
Regional Office for the Americas/Pan American Health Organization
525 23rd Street NW
Washington, DC 20037
Phone: 202-974-3000; 202-974-3457 for the Office of Public Information
Fax: 202-974-3663
Web site: *http://www.who.int*
Founded in 1948, the WHO leads the world alliance for Health for All. A specialized
agency of the United Nations, WHO promotes technical cooperation for health
among nations, carries out programs to control and eradicate disease, and strives to
improve the quality of human life.

International Agency for Research on Cancer (IARC)
World Health Organization
150 cours Albert Thomas
F-69372 Lyon cedex 08, France
Phone: 33-0-4-72-73-84-85
Fax: 33-0-4-72-73-85-75
Web site: *http://www.iarc.fr*
IARC coordinates and conducts research on the causes of human cancer and the
mechanisms of carcinogenesis. The *IARC Monographs*, available on the IARC
Web site, are critical reviews and evaluations of evidence on the carcinogenicity of
a wide range of human exposures. The IARC Web site contains: three databases
with information on the occurrence of cancer worldwide, a database including car-
cinogenic risks to humans, a list of publications, and links to related cancer sites.

Glossary

A

absolute risk: the measured percentage of how a *risk factor* affects the number of cases of *cancer* that occur; used to help avoid overstating the dangers of a risk factor, especially if the risk of something happening is low.

acetone: a poisonous solvent used as a paint stripper and nail polish remover; a component of cigarette smoke.

adenoma: a *benign tumor*; a *polyp*.

adenomatous polyps: small *benign tumors*.

adjuvants: drugs or methods that enhance the effectiveness of medical treatments.

aflatoxin: a *carcinogenic* chemical naturally produced by mold that sometimes contaminates peanuts, wheat, soybeans, ground nuts, corn and rice.

Alar: the trade name for a chemical plant growth regulator used to increase the storage life of fruit; also known as daminozide.

alveoli: tiny grapelike clusters that cover the surface of the lungs and exchange oxygen and carbon dioxide.

Ames test: an *in-vitro* test that shows whether a substance alters *DNA* in bacteria; developed by Bruce N. Ames.

ammonia: a pungent, suffocating gas and a powerful agent used in cleaning; a component of cigarette smoke.

angiogenesis: the process of blood vessel formation.

animal study: the testing of substances on a whole organism in a controlled environment.

antibody: a *protein* produced by the *immune system* in response to infection; each antibody works against a specific *antigen*.

antigens: foreign substances that signal the body's *immune system* to destroy them; substances that when introduced into the body stimulate the production of *antibodies*. Antigens include toxins, bacteria, foreign blood cells, and the cells of transplanted organs.

antioxidants: *nutrients* in fruits and vegetables that appear to protect cells against damage that occurs during normal metabolism; examples include vitamins C and E.

APC: a *tumor suppressor gene*; *mutations* of this *gene* are linked to *familial polyposis*.

apoptosis: normal, programmed cell death.

arsenic: a naturally occurring and highly poisonous metallic element used in pesticides and various alloys; a component of cigarette smoke. Also found in low levels in drinking water.

asbestos: a fibrous mineral used in building and manufacturing as fireproof insulation.

B

BMI: see *body mass index*.

basal cell cancer: *cancer* that begins in the lowest layer of the epidermis called the basal cell layer.

bcr-abl: a *gene* that is linked to *chronic myelogenous leukemia (CML)*. The *bcr-abl* gene expresses the bcr-abl protein.

benzene: a colorless, flammable liquid form from both natural and manmade sources; used chiefly in the manufacture of dyes and as a solvent, it is considered a human *carcinogen*. A component of cigarette smoke.

benign: non-cancerous; not *malignant*.

bioengineered foods: foods made by adding *genes* from other plants or organisms to increase desirable qualities.

biologic therapy: treatment to stimulate or restore the ability of the *immune system* to fight infection and disease.

biomarkers: substances that show up when particular processes are happening in the body.

body mass index (BMI): a ratio of weight in kilograms to height in meters squared; an index of obesity used to determine levels of body fat for adults.

BRCA1: a *tumor suppressor gene*; *mutations* of this *gene* are linked to breast *cancer*.

BRCA2: a *tumor suppressor gene*; *mutations* of this *gene* are linked to breast *cancer*.

butane: a flammable chemical used for lighter fuel and in the manufacturing process of rubber; a component of cigarette smoke.

C

cadmium: a metallic element, found in car batteries; a component of cigarette smoke.

cancer: a group of diseases that cause cells in the body to change and grow out of control.

cancer cluster: the occurrence of a greater than expected number of cases of *cancer* within a group of people, a geographic area, or period of time.

cancer registries: repositories of data that store information about *cancer* detection, diagnosis, stage of disease, treatment, survival, and patient *demographics*.

cancer surveillance: the process of collecting and analyzing information about cancer deaths, new cancer cases, extent of the disease, *screening* tests, treatment, and survival.

cancer vaccine: a preparation that contains *cancer* cells, parts of cells, or pure *antigens*; used to increase the immune response against cancer cells already present in the body.

carbon monoxide: an odorless poisonous gas found in gar exhaust; a component of cigarette smoke.

carcinogen: a *cancer*-causing substance or agent, such as chemicals in tobacco smoke or *ultraviolet radiation*.

carcinogenesis: the process that changes normal cells into cancerous cells.

carcinoma: *malignant tumors* that grow in the tissue that covers or lines the external and internal body surfaces.

carotenoid: a *phytochemical*; an *antioxidant*.

case-control study: a type of *observational study* that looks at the people (or "cases") with a certain type of *cancer* and then compares their histories to those of other people (the "controls") in similar situations who did not develop cancer.

casefinding: identifying people with *cancer* who have sought care at hospitals and doctor's offices.

chemoprevention: the use of natural or laboratory-made substances to reverse, suppress, or prevent cells from developing into *cancer*; not be confused with the prevention of cancer through dietary changes.

chemotherapy: the use of powerful chemicals to treat a disease; in *cancer* medicine, medications that destroy cancer cells.

chromosomes: threadlike bodies in the nucleus of a cell that carry the chemical instructions for reproduction of the cell and transmit *hereditary* information. They consist of strands of *DNA* wrapped in a double helix around a core of *proteins*. Each species of plant or animal has a characteristic number of chromosomes; for example, humans have 46 chromosomes.

chronic myelogenous leukemia (CML): a chronic *malignant* disease in which too many white blood cells are made in the bone marrow; linked to abnormalities in the *bcr-abl* protein.

clinical trial: carefully designed and controlled human research studies that test new ways to treat specific diseases like *cancer*.

CML: see *chronic myelogenous leukemia*.

cohort study: a type of *observational study* that follows a group of people over a period of time.

colonoscope: an optic tube inserted into the rectum that enables a doctor to screen for colon *cancer*.

computed tomography (CT): a radiographic scan in which a three-dimensional image of a body structure is constructed by computer; uses larger doses of *radiation* than an *x-ray*.

congenital: present at birth; can be inherited or caused by environmental factors.

CT: see *computed tomography*.

D

DDT: see *dichloro-diphenyl-trichloro-ethane.*

demographics: characteristics of human populations and population segments such as race, age, ethnicity, and socioeconomic status.

deoxyribonucleic acid (DNA): the cellular material that contains genetic information; the principal constituent of *genes* and *chromosomes.*

DES: see *diethylstilbestrol.*

dichloro-diphenyl-trichloroethane (DDT): a colorless insecticide poisonous to humans and animals. Residue from DDT remains in the ecosystem long after its original use; thus its use is banned in many countries.

dietary supplement: vitamins, minerals, herbs, amino acids, and other products consumed for potential health benefits; dietary supplements are not considered drugs.

diethylstilbestrol (DES): a drug that was prescribed to help prevent miscarriages; no longer prescribed because of the occurrence of reproductive abnormalities and *cancers* in the offspring of women treated with it.

disease cluster: the occurrence of a greater than expected number of cases of a particular disease within a group of people, a geographic area, or period of time.

DNA: see *deoxyribonucleic acid.*

E

ecological study: a type of *observational study* that compares the risk of a disease such as *cancer* in different populations.

electric and magnetic fields (EMF): The field of force associated with electric charge in motion that has electric and magnetic components and contains electromagnetic energy; also called electromagnetic fields.

electromagnetic radiation: a type of *nonionizing radiation* produced by moving electrical charges, found in power lines and electronic devices such as cellular phones and televisions.

EMF: see *electric and magnetic fields.*

environment: the combination of circumstances, physical conditions, and outside influences that surround a person; any factor that is not inherited as part of a person's genetic makeup.

environmental tobacco smoke: cigarette, cigar, or pipe smoke that is inhaled unintentionally by nonsmokers; also called *secondhand smoke.*

epidemiology: the branch of medicine that studies the causes, distribution, and control of disease in populations.

epidemiologist: a scientist who studies the causes, distribution, and control of disease in populations.

ERT: see *estrogen replacement therapy.*

estrogen: a steroid *hormone* responsible for the development and maintenance of female secondary sex characteristics.

estrogen replacement therapy (ERT): the administration of estrogen to relieve symptoms in menopausal women.

F

familial polyposis: any of several inherited diseases that are characterized by the formation of *polyps* in the gastrointestinal tract.

fatty acids: chains of carbon atoms with varying numbers of hydrogen atoms.

fibrocystic breast lumps: *benign* lumps in breast tissue that respond to female *hormones.*

folic acid: a type of vitamin B occurring in green plants, fresh fruit, liver, and yeast.

formaldehyde: a toxic gas used to preserve body tissue; a component of cigarette smoke.

free radical: an atom or group of atoms that has at least one unpaired electron and is therefore highly unstable or reactive; free radicals can damage cells and are believed to accelerate the process of *cancer* and aging.

fungicide: a chemical substance that destroys or inhibits the growth of fungi.

G

gene therapy: the process of inserting a specific *gene* into cells to restore a missing function or to give the cells a new function.

genes: segments of *DNA* that control the expression of traits.

genetic counseling: the counseling of individuals on the probabilities, dangers, diagnosis, and treatment of inherited diseases.

genetic testing: the process of identifying people at risk for developing certain types of disease by checking for *mutations* in inherited *genes*.

genetics: the branch of biology that deals with *heredity*.

genome: the total genetic material contained within an organism. The human genome contains over 30,000 genes.

Gleevec: a drug (trade name: STI571, generic name: imatinib mesylate) that inhibits the abnormal *bcr-abl* protein that seems to be responsible for *chronic myelogenous leukemia (CML)*.

growth factor: a naturally occurring *protein* that causes cells to grow and divide.

H

herbicide: a chemical substance used to destroy or inhibit the growth of plants, especially weeds.

HER2/neu: a *protein* that promotes the growth of *cancer* cells.

Herceptin: a drug (generic name: trastuzumab) that works by preventing the growth of *cancer* cells; a *monoclonal antibody* directed against the *HER2/neu* protein of breast *tumors*.

hereditary: inherited; capable of being transmitted genetically from parent to child.

heredity: the study of the inheritance of traits, variations, and disorders in organisms.

histology: the study of the microscopic structure of animal and plant tissues.

Hodgkin's disease: a *malignant* progressive *cancer* marked by enlargement of the *lymph* nodes, spleen, and liver; also called Hodgkin's lymphoma.

hormone: a chemical substance released by the endocrine glands that travels through the bloodstream to set in motion various body functions.

hormone-replacement therapy (HRT): a combination of the female *hormones* *estrogen* and *progestin* used to relieve symptoms in menopausal women.

HRT: see *hormone-replacement therapy*.

human studies: scientific studies that use human subjects.

hydrogen cyanide: a poisonous gas used to execute prisoners in gas chambers; a component of cigarette smoke.

I

immune system: the complex system that protects the body from foreign substances, cells, and tissues.

immunotherapy: treatment to stimulate or restore the ability of the *immune system* to fight infection and disease; a specific type of *biologic therapy*.

in vitro: in an artificial environment outside a living organism; literally, in glass.

in utero: literally, in the uterus.

incidence rate: the rate of development of new cases of *cancer*.

initiation: the first stage of *carcinogenesis*, in which one or more *oncogenes* or *tumor suppressor genes* are mutated.

initiators: chemicals that triggers cellular changes that can eventually lead to *cancer*; examples include *ultraviolet radiation*, *x-rays*, radon, and many of the chemicals in tobacco smoke.

insecticide: a chemical substance used to kill insects.

interventional study: a study in which researchers intentionally change at least one factor they believe is related to the risk of a disease.

involuntary smoking: the unintentional inhalation of cigarette, cigar, or pipe smoke by nonsmokers; also called *passive smoking*.

ionizing radiation: the emission of energy from a source that can damage *DNA*.

L

laboratory studies: the testing of substances on bacteria, animal, or human cells grown in laboratory dishes or test tubes; also known as test-tube studies.

latency period: the time between exposure to a *carcinogen* and the development of *cancer*.

leukemia: a cancerous disorder of the blood-forming tissues characterized by excessive production of white blood cells.

Li-Fraumeni syndrome: a rare, inherited condition in which patients have a higher risk for developing a variety of cancers.

lifetime risk: the probability that an individual will develop a disease such as *cancer* during his or her lifetime.

lymphatic system: tissues and vessels that create, store, and transport white blood cells to fight infection.

lymph: clear fluid that contains white blood cells.

lymphoma: cancer of the *lymphatic system*. The two main types are *Hodgkin's disease* and *non-Hodgkin's lymphoma*.

M

magnetic resonance imaging (MRI): the use of magnets to produce electronic images of human cells, tissues, and organs.

malignant: cancerous; not *benign*.

mammogram: an *x-ray* of the breast, used to detect breast *cancer*.

medical demography: the statistical study of human populations in order to understand disease patterns.

medical radiation: the emission of energy from diagnostic *x-rays*, *radiation therapy*, and other medical procedures.

melanocytes: pigment-producing cells in the skin.

melanoma: *cancer* that starts in the *melanocytes*.

mesothelioma: a rare *cancer* of the lining of the chest and abdomen associated with exposure to *asbestos*.

metastasis: the spread of *cancer* cells to distant areas of the body by way of the *lymphatic system* or bloodstream.

methanol: a poisonous substance used in solvents, jet engine and rocket fuels, and antifreeze; a component of cigarette smoke.

methylene chloride: a chemical used as a solvent, paint remover, and aerosol propellant.

molecular biology: the branch of science devoted to studying the structure, function, and reactions involved in life processes.

monoclonal antibodies: manmade versions of *immune system proteins* that attach only to a particular target.

monounsaturated fat: a fat whose fatty acid chains are missing two hydrogen atoms, causing the molecules to bend instead of stack, thus becoming a liquid. Olive, peanut, and canola oil are primarily monounsaturated.

morbid anatomy: the study of structural changes in the body that accompany disease; also called *pathological anatomy*.

mouse models: special strains of genetically altered mice used in *cancer* research.

MRI: see *magnetic resonance imaging*.

multistage carcinogenesis: the concept that *cancer* develops in stages.

mutations: changes or mistakes in cells.

N

natural background radiation: the emission of energy from cosmic rays and radioactive elements normally present in soil.

nephroblastoma: a *malignant tumor* of the kidney that primarily affects children; also known as *Wilms' tumor*.

nicotine: a highly addictive and toxic substance that is the active ingredient in many insecticides; a component of cigarette smoke.

nitrosamines: carcinogenic byproducts formed when tobacco is heat dried.

non-Hodgkin's lymphoma: cancer of the lymphatic tissue that is linked to problems with the body's *immune system*.

nonionizing radiation: energy emitted at very low frequencies; does not cause *DNA* damage. Forms of nonionizing radiation include microwaves, radio waves, and radar, as well as *electromagnetic radiation*.

nonmedical synthetic radiation: the emission of energy from aboveground nuclear weapons testing, and occupational and commercial sources.

nonmelanoma: the most common type of skin *cancer*, classified as either *basal cell* or *squamous cell*.

nucleus: the part of the cell that contains *hereditary* material and controls cellular metabolism, growth, and reproduction.

nutrients: compounds found in food (such as carbohydrates, *proteins*, and fats) that are essential to life.

O

obesity: an increase above healthy weight (usually by more than 20 percent) that reduces life expectancy.

observational study: a study that follows real people as they go about their normal lives, without any intervention from researchers; the most common type of epidemiological research.

omega-3 fatty acids: a substance with anticoagulant properties found in animal and vegetable fats and oils; capable of reducing cholesterol levels.

oncogenes: genes that promote cell division; *mutations* in these *genes* may cause the transformation of normal cells into cancerous *tumor* cells.

oncologist: a doctor who specializes in *cancer* treatment.

oncolytic viruses: *viruses* that have *cancer*-killing properties, either naturally or through laboratory manipulation.

P

p53: a *tumor suppressor gene*; *mutations* of this *gene* are linked to more than half of the *cancers* that occur in humans.

paleopathologist: a medical specialist who studies diseases of former times using fossils or other remains.

passive smoking: the unintentional inhalation of cigarette, cigar, or pipe smoke by nonsmokers; also called *involuntary smoking*.

pathological: disease-related.

pathological anatomy: the study of structural changes in the body that accompany disease; also called *morbid anatomy*.

PCBs: see *polychlorinated biphenyls*.

PDT: see *photodynamic therapy*.

pesticide: a chemical substance used to kill pests such as insects, mice and other animals, weeds, fungi, or microorganisms like bacteria and viruses; includes *insecticides, herbicides*, and *fungicides*

PET: see *positron emission tomography*.

phenoxy herbicides: a group of highly poisonous chemical substances used to destroy or inhibit the growth of plants, especially weeds.

phenylketonuria: a disorder in which an individual is unable to metabolize the naturally occurring amino acid phenylalanine, a chemical found in the artificial sweetener aspartame.

photodynamic therapy (PDT): a treatment that combines a light source and a *photosensitizing agent* to destroy *cancer* cells. Also called photoradiation therapy, phototherapy, or photochemotherapy.

photosensitizing agent: a drug activated by light.

phytochemicals: plant substances considered to have a beneficial effect on human health.

placebo: an inactive substance used as a control in an experiment to determine the effectiveness of a medicinal drug; a dummy pill that has no effect.

polonium-210: a highly radioactive element; a component of cigarette smoke.

polychlorinated biphenyls (PCBs): a group of more than 200 industrial chemicals used in industry until they were banned by Congress in 1976 due to concerns about toxicity and environmental impact.

polyps: *benign tumors*; projectile growths of tissue into the center of the colon or rectum.

polyunsaturated fat: a fat whose fatty acid chains are missing many hydrogen atoms, causing the molecules bend in several places, making them liquid. Most vegetable oils and fish oils are primarily polyunsaturated.

positron emission tomography (PET): a medical imaging technique that measures cellular activity by tracking the movement and concentration of a radioactive tracer that is injected into the body. The technique requires special computerized imaging equipment.

preventive surgery: surgery performed to preventing or slowing the course of an illness or disease; also called prophylactic surgery.

progestin: a female steroid sex *hormone*.

progression: the third stage of *carcinogenesis*, in which *cancer* cells may grow, become more aggressive, and metastasize.

promoters: chemicals that lead cells to become cancerous; examples include bile acids and *estrogens*.

promotion: the second stage of *carcinogenesis*, in which the cells damaged by *initiators* grow.

prophylactic: preventative.

protein: an essential nutrient found in foods such as meat, fish, eggs, and beans; required for human growth and tissue repair. Proteins are large molecules made up of a chain of smaller units called amino acids that serve many vital functions.

proto-oncogenes: genes that help a cell grow and divide normally.

R

RB: a *tumor suppressor gene*; mutations of this *gene* are linked to *retinoblastoma*.

rad: a unit of radiation dose.

radiation: the emission of energy from a source.

radiation therapy: the medical use of high-energy *ionizing radiation* to destroy *cancer* cells and treat or control cancer.

radioactive decay: the natural breakdown of a radioactive atom which releases *ionizing radiation*.

radon: a colorless, odorless gas that occurs naturally in soil, rocks, underground water, and air; a known cause of lung cancer.

randomized controlled clinical trial: an *interventional study* in which people are randomly assigned to one group or another, and some factor is intentionally kept different between the two groups.

relative risk: a measure of how strongly a *risk factor* influences the development of *cancer*; used to give a sense of what will happen if one person is exposed to a risk factor and another is not.

remission: a disease-free period.

retinoblastoma: a rare *hereditary malignant tumor* of the eye, occurring chiefly in young children.

rhabdomyosarcoma (RMS): a *cancer* that affects the skeletal muscles, found primarily in children. The most common soft-tissue childhood cancer.

RMS: see *rhabdomyosarcoma*.

risk factor: anything that increases a person's chance of getting a disease.

S

sarcoma: *malignant tumors* that grow in the connective tissues.

saturated fat: a fat whose fatty acid chains are loaded, or saturated, with hydrogen atoms; saturated fats are usually solid at room temperature, and are found in butter, red meat, poultry, milk products, and certain "tropical" vegetable oils such as palm kernel and coconut oils.

schistosomiasis: a disease caused by infestation with parasitic worms called flukes, through use of contaminated water, and characterized by infection and gradual destruction of the tissues of the kidneys, liver, and other organs.

screening: the search for disease, such as *cancer*, in people without symptoms.

secondhand smoke: cigarette, cigar, or pipe smoke that is inhaled unintentionally by nonsmokers; also called *environmental tobacco smoke*.

selenium: a nonmetallic chemical element; an *antioxidant*.

SPF: see *sun protection factor*.

sporadic cancer: non-inherited *cancer*.

squamous cell cancer: *cancer* that begins in the higher levels of the epidermis.

statistical significance: a measurement used to describe how often a particular result would occur simply by chance if a study or experiment were repeated many times. The most common minimal level accepted for statistical significance is 95 percent, meaning that if the study were repeated many times, the probability of the same result occurring due to chance alone would be 5 percent or less.

sun protection factor (SPF): The degree to which a sunscreen, suntan lotion, or similar preparation protects the skin from ultraviolet rays, usually expressed numerically. SPF 15, for example, will provide 15 times the protection of no sunscreen.

T

talc: a mineral powder used for medicinal and toiletry products.

tamoxifen: a drug (trade name Nolvadex) used as *hormone* therapy to treat advanced breast *cancer* in women whose tumors are *estrogen*-dependent; also used *prophylactically* by some women at risk for breast cancer.

telomerase: an enzyme that encourages cells to keep dividing indefinitely instead of dying with age; thought to be an element in the development of human *cancers*.

toluene: a poisonous industrial solvent, also used in the manufacture of explosives; a component of cigarette smoke.

trans fat: a fat that has undergone a food-industry process called hydrogenation that adds hydrogen to an unsaturated fat, such as vegetable oil, resulting in straight molecules that stack into a semi-solid, making it spreadable like margarine.

tumor: an abnormal mass of tissue; can be *benign* or *malignant*.

tumor suppressor genes: genes that prevent cells from dividing too quickly; they also send messages to tell cells when to repair damage to *DNA* or to die.

U

UV Index: a measure of the damaging potential of *ultraviolet (UV) radiation* reaching the earth's surface around noon each day.

UVA rays: energy that travels from the sun that is not absorbed by the ozone layer; one of three wavelength categories of *ultraviolet (UV) radiation*. UVA rays are involved in the aging of cells and some damage to *DNA*.

UVB rays: energy that travels from the sun that is partially absorbed by the ozone layer; one of three wavelength categories of *ultraviolet (UV) radiation*. UVB rays cause direct damage to *DNA* and are thought to cause most skin *cancers*.

UVC rays: energy that travels from the sun that is absorbed by the ozone layer and does not reach earth; one of three wavelength categories of *ultraviolet (UV) radiation*. UVC rays pose no risk to humans.

ultrasound: The use of sound waves to image an internal body structure.

ultraviolet (UV) radiation: the emission of energy from sunlight or artificial tanning machines; the cause of almost all cases of skin *cancer*.

V

vaccine: a preparation that uses weakened or killed *viruses*, bacteria, or other germs to prevent infectious diseases in healthy people.

viruses: very small disease-causing organisms unable to reproduce without a host cell.

vitamin C: an *antioxidant* found in fruits and leafy vegetables or made synthetically; also called ascorbic acid.

vitamin E: an *antioxidant* found in plant leaves, wheat germ oil, and milk.

W

Wilms' tumor: A *malignant tumor* of the kidney that primarily affects children; also known as *nephroblastoma*.

X

x-ray: one form of *radiation* that can be used at low levels to produce an image of the body on film or at high levels to destroy *cancer* cells.

References

Chapter 1

Adams, S. H. 1913. "What Can We Do About Cancer?" *The Ladies' Home Journal* (May).

American Institute for Cancer Research/World Cancer Research Fund. 1997. *Food, Nutrition and the Prevention of Cancer: A Global Perspective.* Washington, D.C.

Ames, Bruce N., Lois Swirsky Gold, and Walter C. Willett. 1995. "The Causes and Prevention of Cancer." *Proceedings of the National Academy of Sciences of the United States of America* 92 (12):5258–5265 (6 June).

Dodson, J. Lynne. 1997. *A Century of Oncology: A Photographic History of Cancer Research and Therapy.* Greenwich Press: Greenwich, Connecticut.

Doll, Richard. 1998. "Uncovering the Effects of Smoking: Historical Perspective." *Statistical Methods in Medical Research* 7 (2):87–117 (June).

Doll, Richard and Richard Peto. 1981. "The Causes of Cancer: Quantitative Estimates of Avoidable Risks of Cancer in the United States Today." *Journal of the National Cancer Institute* 66 (6):1191–1308 (June).

Heath, Clark W., Jr., and Elizabeth T. H. Fontham. 2001. Cancer Etiology. Chap. 3 in *Clinical Oncology.* Edited by Raymond E. Lenhard, Jr., Robert T. Osteen, and Ted Gansler. Atlanta, Georgia: American Cancer Society.

National Cancer Institute. "Closing In On Cancer: Solving a 5,000-Year-Old Mystery." Available at: *http://press2.nci.nih.gov/sciencebehind/cioc/ciocframe.htm.*

Pott, Percivall. 1775. Cancer scroti. Pages 63–68 in *Chirurgical Observations Relative to the Cataract, the Polypus of the Nose, the Cancer of the Scrotum, the Different Kinds of Ruptures, and the Mortification of the Toes and Feet.* London: Printed by T.J. Carnegy for L. Hawes, W. Clarke and R.Collins.

Shimkin, Michael B. 1977. *Contrary to Nature: Being an Illustrated Commentary on Some Persons and Events of Historical Importance in the Development of Knowledge Concerning...Cancer.* U.S. Department of Health, Education, and Welfare, Public Health Service, National Institutes of Health. Washington: U.S. Government Printing Office.

United States Department of Health and Human Services, Centers for Disease Control and Prevention, National Center for Infectious Diseases, Division of Parasitic Diseases. "Fact Sheet: Schistosomiasis." Available at: *http://www.cdc.gov/ncidod/dpd/parasites/schistosomiasis/factsht_schistosomiasis.htm*

World Health Organization. 1996. "Schistosomiasis." Fact Sheet No. 115. Available at: *http://www.who.int/inf-fs/en/fact115.html.*

Chapter 2

American Cancer Society. 2002. *Cancer Control State-of-the-Science Guide.* Atlanta, Georgia: ACS Publication.

American Cancer Society. 2000. *Cancer Facts and Figures for African Americans, 2000–2001.* Atlanta, Georgia: ACS Publication.

American Cancer Society. 2000. *Cancer Facts and Figures for Hispanics, 2000–2001.* Atlanta, Georgia: ACS Publication.

American Cancer Society. 1989. "A Summary of the American Cancer Society Report to the Nation: Cancer in the Poor." *CA: A Cancer Journal for Clinicians* 39 (5):263–265 (September/October).

American Cancer Society. 2002. "The African-American Cancer Burden: Researcher Attacks High Cancer Rates with Science." Available at: *http://www.cancer.org/docroot/SPC/content/SPC_1_Jones_Lovell_On_African_American_Cancer_Rates.asp.*

00

American Cancer Society. 2002. "Some Ethnic Groups May Have More Aggressive Breast Cancers: Reasons Are Unclear." ACS News Today (12 August). Available at: *http://www.cancer.org/docroot/NWS/content/NWS_1_1x_Some_Ethnic_Groups_May_Have_More_Aggressive_Breast_Cancers.asp*.

Anderson, Robert N. 2002. United States Department of Health and Human Services, Centers for Disease Control and Prevention, National Center for Health Statistics, Division of Vital Statistics. "Deaths: Leading Causes for 2000." *National Vital Statistics Reports* 50 (16): 86 pages (16 September).

Brawley, Otis W. 2002. "Some Perspectives on Black-White Cancer Statistics." *CA: A Cancer Journal for Clinicians* 52 (6):322–325 (November/December).

Brawley, Otis W., and Harold P. Freeman. 1999. "Race and Outcomes: Is This the End of the Beginning for Minority Health Research?" *Journal of the National Cancer Institute* 91 (22):1908–1909.

Cohen, Harvey Jay. 1999. Oncology and Aging: General Principles of Cancer in the Elderly. Chapter 8 in *Principles of Geriatric Medicine and Gerontology*, 4th ed. Edited by William R. Hazzard et al. New York: McGraw-Hill.

Deapen, Dennis, et al. 2002. "Rapidly Rising Breast Cancer Incidence Rates Among Asian-American Women." *International Journal of Cancer* 99 (5):747–750 (10 June).

Freeman, Harold P. 1989. "Cancer in the Socioeconomically Disadvantaged." *CA: A Cancer Journal for Clinicians* 39 (5):266–288 (September/October).

Henschke U. K. et al. 1973. "Alarming Increase of the Cancer Mortality in the U.S. Black Population (1950–1967)." *Cancer* 31 (4):763–768 (April).

Hunter, Carrie P., Karen A. Johnson, and Hyman B. Muss. 2000. *Cancer in the Elderly*. New York: Marcel Dekker.

Intercultural Cancer Council. 2001. "Cancer Fact Sheets." Available at: *http://iccnetwork.org/cancerfacts*.

Kennedy, B. J. 2000. "Aging and Cancer." *Oncology* 14 (12):1731–1740 (December).

Li, Christopher I., Kathleen E. Malone, and Janet R. Daling. 2002. "Differences in Breast Cancer Hormone Receptor Status and Histology by Race and Ethnicity among Women 50 Years of Age and Older." *Cancer Epidemiology, Biomarkers and Prevention* 11 (7):601–607 (July).

McPhee, S. J. 2002. "Caring for a 70-year-old Vietnamese Woman." *Journal of the American Medical Association* 287 (4):495–504.

Newman, Lisa et al. 2002. "African American Ethnicity, Socioeconomic Status, and Breast Cancer Survival." *Cancer* 94 (11):2844–2854 (May).

Ross, Houkje. 2000. "Lay Health Workers Can Help Change Behaviors." *Closing the Gap, A Newsletter of the Office of Minority Health*, U.S. Department of Health and Human Services (August): 7.

United States Census Bureau. 2001. "The White Population: 2000." Available at: *http://www.census.gov/prod/2001pubs/c2kbr01-4.pdf*.

United States Census Bureau. 2002. "The Asian Population: 2000." Available at: *http://www.census.gov/prod/2002pubs/c2kbr01-16.pdf*.

United States Census Bureau. 2001. "The Black Population: 2000." Available at: *http://www.census.gov/prod/2001pubs/c2kbr01-5.pdf*.

United States Census Bureau. 2001. "The Hispanic Population: 2000." Available at: *http://www.census.gov/prod/2001pubs/c2kbr01-3.pdf*.

United States Census Bureau. 2002. "Poverty in the United States: 2001." Available at: *http://www.census.gov/prod/2002pubs/p60-219.pdf*.

Weinberg, Robert A. *1998. One Renegade Cell: How Cancer Begins*. New York: Basic Books.

Wingo, Phyllis A., Donald M. Parkin, and Harmon J. Eyre. 2001. Measuring the Occurrence of Cancer: Impact and Statistics. Chap. 1 in *Clinical Oncology*. Edited by Raymond E. Lenhard, Jr., Robert T. Osteen, and Ted Gansler. Atlanta, Georgia: American Cancer Society.

Chapter 3

American Cancer Society. 2002. *Good for You! Reducing Your Risk of Developing Cancer*. Atlanta, Georgia: American Cancer Society.

American College of Surgeons. 1997. *AJCC Cancer Staging Manual/American Joint Committee on Cancer*, 5th ed. Edited by Irvin D. Fleming et al. Philadelphia: Lippincott-Raven.

Bishop, Jerry E. and Michael Waldholz. 1990. *Genome: The Story of the Most Astonishing Scientific Adventure of Our Time–The Attempt to Map All the Genes in the Human Body*. New York: Simon and Schuster.

Clarke, Karen M. 2001. "Breast Cancer Genetics in Primary Care." *Physicians Assistant* 25 (10):20–28 (October).

Cline, Robin. 1999. "Knudson Gives NCI Partners in Research Lecture." *The NIH Record* 51 (18) (7 September). Available at: *http://www.nih.gov/news/NIH-Record/09_07_99/story03.htm*.

Eyre, Harmon J., Dianne Partie Lange, and Lois B. Morris. 2001. *Informed Decisions: The Complete Book of Cancer Diagnosis, Treatment, and Recovery*, 2nd ed. Atlanta, Georgia: American Cancer Society.

Fox Chase Cancer Center. 2002. "Fox Chase Cancer Center's Alfred G. Knudson Honored with 2002 Special Award from ASCO" (20 May). Available at: *http://www.fccc.edu/news/2002/Knudson-Award-05-20-2002.html*.

Li, Frederick P., and Joseph F. Fraumeni, Jr. 1969. "Rhabdomyosarcoma in Children: Epidemiologic Study and Identification of a Familial Cancer Syndrome." *Journal of the National Cancer Institute* 43 (6):1365–1373 (December).

Rubin, Philip, ed. 1993. *Clinical Oncology for Medical Students and Physicians: A Multi-disciplinary Approach*, 7th ed. Philadelphia: W.B. Saunders Company.

Schottenfeld, David, and Joseph F. Fraumeni, Jr., ed. 1996. *Cancer Epidemiology and Prevention*, 2d ed. New York: Oxford University Press.

Weber, Barbara L. 1996. "Genetic Testing for Breast Cancer." *Scientific American Science and Medicine* 3 (1):12–21 (January/February).

Weinberg, Robert A. 1998. *One Renegade Cell: How Cancer Begins*. New York: Basic Books.

Chapter 4

American Cancer Society. 2002. *Good for You! Reducing Your Risk of Developing Cancer*. Atlanta, Georgia: American Cancer Society.

American Cancer Society. 2001. *Breast Cancer Facts and Figures, 2001–2002*. Atlanta, Georgia: ACS Publication.

American Cancer Society. 1999. "Making Sense of Scientific Studies: Questions to Ask." ACS News Today (25 January). Available at: *http://www.cancer.org/docroot/NWS/content/NWS_3_1x_Making_Sense_of_Scientific_Studies__Questions_to_A.asp*

Department of Health and Human Services, National Institutes of Health, National Cancer Institute. 2002. "How To Evaluate Health Information on the Internet:

Questions and Answers." Cancer Facts 2.10 (28 August). Available at: *http://cis.nci.nih.gov/fact/2_10.htm*.

Frumkin, Howard, et al. 2001. "Cellular Phones and Risk of Brain Tumors." *CA: A Cancer Journal for Clinicians* 51 (2):137–141 (March/April).

Godoy, Maria. 2000. "Does Science Support Cell Phone-Cancer Connection?" (3 August). Available at: *http://www.techtv.com/news/politicsandlaw/story/0,24195,3698,00.html*.

Malenka, David J., et al. 1993. "The Framing Effect of Relative and Absolute Risk." *Journal of General Internal Medicine* 8(10): 543–548 (October).

Marshall, Eliot. 1991. "A is for Apple, Alar and...Alarmist?" *Science* 254 (5028):20–22 (4 October).

Murray, David, Joel Schwartz, and S. Robert Lichter. 2001. *It Ain't Necessarily So: How Media Make and Unmake the Scientific Picture of Reality*. Lanham, Maryland: Rowman and Littlefield Publishers.

Newman, Chris, John Moulder, David Reynard, and David Feigal. 2000. "Do Cell Phones Cause Cancer?" Interview by Larry King. *Larry King Live*. CNN, 9 August. Also available at: *http://www.sarshield.com/news/stories/cellphonecausecancer.html*.

Nordenberg, Tamar. 2000. "Cell Phones and Brain Cancer: No Clear Connection." *FDA Consumer* 34 (6) (November/December). Available at: *http://www.fda.gov/fdac/features/2000/600_phone.html*.

Paulos, John Allen. 1996. *A Mathematician Reads the Newspaper*. New York: Anchor Books.

Ross, John F. 1995. "Risk: Where Do Real Dangers Lie?" *Smithsonian* (November). Available at: *http://www.smithsonianmag.si.edu/smithsonian/issues95/nov95/risk_nov95.html*

Sharp, Richard, et al. 2002. "Synergism Between INK4a/ARF Inactivation and Aberrant HGF/SF Signaling in Rhabdomyosarcomagenesis." *Nature Medicine* 8: 1276–1280 (1 November).

Willett, Walter C. 2001. *Eat, Drink and Be Healthy: The Harvard Medical School Guide to Healthy Eating*. New York: Simon and Schuster.

Woloshin, Steven, Lisa M. Schwartz, and H. Gilbert Welch. 2002. "Risk Charts: Putting Cancer in Context." *Journal of the National Cancer Institute* 94 (11):799–804 (June).

Chapter 5

American Cancer Society. 2002. "Breast Cancer on Long Island: Experts Find Some Answers, Seek More." ACS News Today (9 October). Available at: *http://www.cancer.org/docroot/NWS/content/NWS_1_1x_Breast_Cancer_On_Long_Island_Researchers_Find_Some_Answers_Seek_More.asp.*

American Cancer Society. 2002. "Florida Program Promotes Skin Cancer Awareness." ACS News Today (18 May). Available at: *http://www.cancer.org/docroot/NWS/content/NWS_5_1x_Florida_Teacher_Shows_Kids_a_Future_Without_Skin_Cancer.asp.*

American Cancer Society. 2002. *Good for You! Reducing Your Risk of Developing Cancer.* Atlanta, Georgia: American Cancer Society.

American Cancer Society. 2002. "Hormone Replacement Therapy: Friend or Foe?" (27 September). Available at: *http://www.cancer.org/docroot/spc/content/spc_1_hrt_explainer_2002.asp.*

American Cancer Society. 2002. "A Pretty Tan Can Leave a Deadly Legacy." ACS News Today (1 July). Available at: *http://www.cancer.org/docroot/NWS/content/NWS_3_1x_Making_Sense_of_Scientific_Studies__Questions_to_A.asp.*

American Cancer Society. 2002. "Sun Exposure." *Cancer Prevention and Early Detection: Facts and Figures 2002,* pp. 22–23. Atlanta, Georgia: ACS Publication.

American Cancer Society. 2001. "Chemical Pollutants: No Link to Breast Cancer." ACS News Today (13 June). Available at: *http://www.cancer.org/docroot/NWS/content/NWS_1_1xU_Chemical_Pollutants__No_Link_to_Breast_Cancer_.asp.*

American Cancer Society. 1999. "Do Pesticides and Dry Cleaning Solvents Affect Breast Cancer Risk?" ACS News Today (22 October). Available at: *http://www.cancer.org/docroot/NWS/content/NWS_1_1x_Do_Pesticides_and_Dry_Cleaning_Solvents_Affect_Breast_Cancer_Risk_.asp.*

American Cancer Society. 1998. "Cancer Clusters Hard to Prove." ACS News Today (18 November). Available at: *http://www.cancer.org/docroot/NWS/content/NWS_1_1x_Cancer_Clusters_Hard_to_Prove.asp.*

American Cancer Society. 1998. "Green World: Work, Home, and Play Can Affect Your Health." ACS News Today (2 November). Available at: *http://www.cancer.org/docroot/NWS/content/NWS_2_1x_Green_World.asp.*

Department of Health and Human Services, National Institutes of Health, National Cancer Institute, Cancer Information Service. 2001. "Cancer Clusters." Cancer Facts 3.58 (19 November). Available at: *http://cis.nci.nih.gov/fact/3_58.htm.*

Department of Health and Human Services, National Institutes of Health, National Cancer Institute. 2002. "Plans and Priorities for Cancer Research: The Nation's Investment in Cancer Research for Fiscal Year 2004." (October). NIH Publication No. 03-4373.

Fagin, Dan. 2002. "'No Closed Doors' on Cancer Research: Activists to Push Studies on Toxins, Breast Cancer Link." Newsday (7 August). Available at: *http://www.newsday.com/news/local/longisland/ny-licanc0807.story.*

Fagin, Dan. 2002. "Tattered Hopes: A $30-Million Federal Study of Breast Cancer and Pollution on LI Has Disappointed Activists and Scientists." Newsday (28 July). Available at: *http://www.newsday.com/news/health/ny-licanc0728.story.*

Fox Chase Cancer Center. 2002. "Non-melanoma Skin Cancer." Available at: *http://www.fccc.edu/clinical/skin/non-melanoma.*

Gammon, Marilie D., et al. 2002. "Environmental Toxins and Breast Cancer on Long Island. I. Polycyclic Aromatic Hydrocarbon DNA Adducts." *Cancer Epidemiology Biomarkers and Prevention* 11 (8):677–685 (August).

Gammon, Marilie D., et al. 2002. "Environmental Toxins and Breast Cancer on Long Island. II. Organochlorine Compound Levels in Blood." *Cancer Epidemiology Biomarkers and Prevention* 11 (8):686–697 (August).

Heimlich, Joe E. 1998. "The Invisible Environment Series: PCBs." Ohio State University Extension Community Development Fact Sheet CDFS-201-98. Available at: *http://ohioline.osu.edu/cd-fact/0201.html.*

Nesmith, Jeff. 2002. Toxins in Air Raise Cancer Risk. *The Atlanta Journal-Constitution,* 1 June:A1.

Nevada State Health Division. 2002. "Leukemia Cluster: Churchill County (Fallon) Childhood Leukemia Update." (20 August). Available at: *http://health2k.state.nv.us/HealthOfficer/Leukemia/Fallon.htm.*

Reno Gazette-Journal. 2002. "A Measure of Fear: The Chronology of the Fallon Cancer Cluster" (26 August). Available at:

http://www.rgj.com/news/stories/html/2002/06/04/15968.php?sp1=&sp2=&sp3=.

Savitz, D. A., and D. P. Loomis. 1995. "Magnetic Field Exposure in Relation to Leukemia and Brain Cancer Mortality Among Electric Utility Workers." *American Journal of Epidemiology* 141 (2):123–134 (15 January). [Erratum published in the 1996 *American Journal of Epidemiology* 144 (2):205 (15 July)].

United States Department of Health and Human Services, Centers for Disease Control and Prevention, National Center for Environmental Health, Division of Environmental Hazards and Health Effects. 2002. "CDC's Role in Investigating Cancer Clusters." (October) Atlanta, Georgia: NCEH Publication No. 02-0594. Also available at: *http://www.cdc.gov/nceh/clusters/CDC%20cluster%20role.htm.*

United States Environmental Protection Agency. 2002. "Polychlorinated Biphenyls (PCBs)." PCB home page at EPA. Available at: *http://www.epa.gov/opptintr/pcb.*

Chapter 6

American Cancer Society. 2002. *Good for You! Reducing Your Risk of Developing Cancer.* Atlanta, Georgia: American Cancer Society.

American Cancer Society. 2001. "EPA Cuts Allowable Arsenic Level in Water." ACS News Today (31 January). Available at: *http://www.cancer.org/docroot/NWS/content/NWS_1_1x_EPA_Cuts_Allowable_Arsenic_Level_in_Water_.asp.*

American Cancer Society. 2001. "Nuclear Weapons Workers May Qualify for New Federal Benefits: Thousands Exposed to Radiation, Beryllium, Silica." ACS News Today (16 October). Available at: *http://www.cancer.org/docroot/NWS/content/NWS_1_1x_Nuclear_Weapons_Workers_May_Qualify_for_New_Federal_Benefits.asp.*

Business Publishers, Inc. 2002. *Clean Water Report* 40 (12) (17 June).

Frumkin, Howard, and Michael J. Thun. 2001. "Arsenic." *CA: A Cancer Journal for Clinicians* 51 (4):254–262 (July/August).

Mirick, Dana K., Scott Davis, and David B. Thomas. 2002. "Antiperspirant Use and the Risk of Breast Cancer." *Journal of the National Cancer Institute* 94 (20):1578–1580 (16 October 16).

Saccharin Warning Elimination via Environmental Testing Employing Science and Technology (SWEETEST) Act. 2000. U. S.

House. 106th Cong., 2d sess., H.R. 5668 IH. (15 December 2000).

United States Department of Health and Human Services, Centers for Disease Control and Prevention, National Institute for Occupational Safety and Health. 2002. "Occupational Cancer." Available at: *http://www.cdc.gov/niosh/occancer.html.*

United States Environmental Protection Agency, Office of Ground Water and Drinking Water. 1998. "Consumer Confidence Reports: Final Rule." Washington, D.C.: EPA Publication No. EPA-816-F-98-007 (August). Also available at: *http://www.epa.gov/safewater/ccr/ccrfact.html.*

United States Environmental Protection Agency, Office of Pesticide Programs. 1998. "Pesticides and Food: What You and Your Family Need to Know." Washington, D.C.: EPA Publication No. EPA-735-F-98-001. Also available at: *http://www.epa.gov/pesticides/food.*

Chapter 7

American Cancer Society. 2003. *Kicking Butts: Quit Smoking and Take Charge of Your Health.* Atlanta, Georgia: American Cancer Society.

American Cancer Society. 2002. *Good for You! Reducing Your Risk of Developing Cancer.* Atlanta, Georgia: American Cancer Society.

American Cancer Society. 2002. "Too Much Insulin May Make Breast Cancer Worse: Obese Women Tend to Have More Insulin." ACS News Today (21 March). Available at: *http://www.cancer.org/docroot/NWS/content/NWS_1_1x_Too_Much_Insulin_May_Make_Breast_Cancer_Worse.asp.*

American Cancer Society. 2001. "Lung Cancer Takes High Toll on African Americans: Researcher Urges Increased Focus on Understanding Lung Cancer in African Americans." ACS News Today (20 July). Available at: *http://www.cancer.org/docroot/NWS/content/NWS_1_1xU_Lung_Cancer_Takes_High_Toll_on_African_Americans.asp.*

American Cancer Society. 2001. "WHO Calls for Worldwide Ban on Public Smoking." ACS News Today (19 June). Available at: *http://www.cancer.org/docroot/NWS/content/update/NWS_1_1xU_WHO_Calls_for_Worldwide_Ban_on_Public_Smoking.asp.*

American Cancer Society. 1999. *Cooking Smart*. Atlanta, Georgia: ACS Publication No. 2642.01.

American Cancer Society. 2002. *Living Smart: The American Cancer Society's Guide to Eating Healthy and Being Active.* Atlanta, Georgia: ACS Publication No. 2042.00.

American Institute for Cancer Research/World Cancer Research Fund. 1997. *Food, Nutrition and the Prevention of Cancer: A Global Perspective*. Washington, D.C.

American Lung Association. 2002. "Tobacco Control." Tobacco Control home page. Available at: *http://www.lungusa.org/tobacco*.

Byers, Tim, et al. 2002. "American Cancer Society Guidelines on Nutrition and Physical Activity for Cancer Prevention: Reducing the Risk of Cancer with Healthy Food Choices and Physical Activity." *CA: A Cancer Journal for Clinicians* 52 (2):92–119 (March/April).

CNN.com. "Focus: Tobacco Under Attack: A Brief History of Tobacco." Available at: *http://www.cnn.com/US/9705/tobacco/history/index.html*.

Doll, Richard. 1998. "Uncovering the Effects of Smoking: Historical Perspective." *Statistical Methods in Medical Research* 7 (2):87–117 (June).

Hoffmann, Dietrich, and Ilse Hoffmann. 1997. "The Changing Cigarette, 1950–1995." *Journal of Toxicology and Environmental Health* 50 (4): 307–364 (March).

Lahey Clinic Health Magazine Special Women's Health Issue. 1998. "The Debate on Dietary Fat." Available at: *http://www.lahey.org/media/healet/Women1998/Dietary_Fat.stm*.

United States Department of Health and Human Services, Centers for Disease Control and Prevention, National Center for Chronic Disease and Health Promotion, Office on Smoking and Health. 1994 and 1996. "History of the 1964 Surgeon General's Report on Smoking and Health." (Compiled January 1994 and July 1996). Available at: *http://www.cdc.gov/tobacco/30yrsgen.htm*.

United States Department of Health and Human Services, Centers for Disease Control. 2002. "Cigarette Smoking Among Adults—United States, 2000." *Morbidity and Mortality Weekly Report* 51 (29):642–645 (26 July).

United States Department of Health and Human Services, Public Health Service, Centers for Disease Control and Prevention, Center for Chronic Disease Prevention and Health Promotion, Office on Smoking and Health. 1989. "Reducing the Health Consequences of Smoking: 25 Years of Progress: A Report of the Surgeon General." DHHS Publication No. (CDC) 89-8411. Rockville, Maryland: U.S. Government Printing Office.

United States Department of Health and Human Services, Centers for Disease Control and Prevention, National Center for Chronic Disease Prevention and Health Promotion, Office on Smoking and Health. 2000. "Reducing Tobacco Use: A Report of the Surgeon General." Atlanta, Georgia: USDHHS publication.

Willett, Walter C. 2002. "Harvesting the Fruits of Research: New Guidelines on Nutrition and Physical Activity." *CA: A Cancer Journal for Clinicians* 52 (2):66–67 (March/April).

Willett, Walter C. 2001. *Eat, Drink and Be Healthy: The Harvard Medical School Guide to Healthy Eating*. New York: Simon and Schuster.

Conclusion

Abbott, Alison. 2002. "On the Offensive." *Nature* 416 (6880):470–474 (4 April).

American Cancer Society. 2002. *Cancer Control State-of-the-Science Guide*. Atlanta, Georgia: ACS Publication.

Department of Health and Human Services, National Institutes of Health, National Cancer Institute. 2002. "Plans and Priorities for Cancer Research: The Nation's Investment in Cancer Research for Fiscal Year 2004." (October). NIH Publication No. 03-4373.

Department of Health and Human Services, National Institutes of Health, National Cancer Institute. 2001. "Cancer Progress Report 2001." Publication No. T905. Available at: *http://progressreport.cancer.gov*.

Eyre, Harmon J. "Cancer in the New Century." Health Resource Center: Fall Health and Fitness 2002. Newsweek.com. Available at: *http://www.washingtonpost.com/wp-adv/newsweek/fall_health_article11.html*.

Weinberg, Robert A. *1998. One Renegade Cell: How Cancer Begins*. New York: Basic Books.

Index